HELP FOR THE
HARD-OF-HEARING

HELP FOR THE
HARD-OF-HEARING

A Speech Reading and Auditory Training Manual for
Home and Professionally Guided Training

By

OLAF HAUG, Ph.D.

Director, Audiology and Vestibular Department
Medical Center Ear, Nose and Throat Associates
Clinical Assistant Professor of Audiology and Speech Pathology
Department of Otolaryngology
Baylor College of Medicine
Houston, Texas

and

SCOTT HAUG, M.A.

Audiology and Vestibulography Department
Austin Ear, Nose and Throat Clinic
Austin, Texas

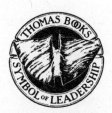

CHARLES C THOMAS • PUBLISHER
Springfield • Illinois • U.S.A.

Published and Distributed Throughout the World by

CHARLES C THOMAS ● PUBLISHER

Bannerstone House

301-327 East Lawrence Avenue, Springfield, Illinois, U.S.A.

© *1977, by* CHARLES C THOMAS ● PUBLISHER

ISBN 0-398-03674-8 (cloth)
ISBN 0-398-03675-6 (paper)

Library of Congress Catalog Card Number: 77-4482

With THOMAS BOOKS *careful attention is given to all details of
manufacturing and design. It is the Publisher's desire to present books that
are satisfactory as to their physical qualities and artistic possibilities and
appropriate for their particular use.* THOMAS BOOKS *will be true to those
laws of quality that assure a good name and good will.*

Printed in the United States of America

R-1

Library of Congress Cataloging in Publication Data

Haug, Olaf.
  Help for the hard-of-hearing.

  Bibliography: p.
  Includes index.
  1. Deaf--Rehabilitation--Handbooks, manuals, etc.
2. Deaf--Means of communication--Handbooks, manuals,
etc. 3. Lipreading--Handbooks, manuals, etc. 4. Hearing aids. I. Haug, Scott, joint author. II. Title.
HV2395.H38   362.4'2   77-4482
ISBN 0-398-03674-8
ISBN 0-398-03675-6 pbk.

PREFACE

THE purpose of this book is to present a simple, practical, clinically proven home training program for the development of speech reading and auditory training skills to help the hard-of-hearing adult or child achieve the maximum benefit from his hearing aid. In addition, it is designed to help the hard-of-hearing person with a loss too slight or too severe for hearing aid benefit. This individual may improve his speech understanding by learning to interpret visual communication cues and by learning to make more meaning out of speech sounds which are perceived by his impaired ears as being weak, imperfect, or distorted.

The book may be used as a guide or framework for a professionally directed auditory habilitation or rehabilitation program. Physicians (particularly the ear, nose, and throat specialists), audiologists, deaf educators, and speech pathologists should find this material very helpful in working with the hearing impaired.

This work is a distillation of a combined thirty-five years of authors' experience in counseling and teaching better speech understanding skills, to the deaf or partially hearing, in a private audiological setting. The methods and suggestions discussed were developed and perfected in training sessions dealing directly with hard-of-hearing patients or through outlining and following up prescribed home training programs.

Some of the unique or outstanding features of the book are as follows:

1. Helps the reader gain a better overall insight into his or her particular communication problem by providing a table which, when filled in by the physician or audiologist, gives a specific detailed description of the patient's hearing loss and communication problems.

2. Provides a simple, practical, but comprehensive discussion of hearing aid care, maintenance, and troubleshooting, including such things as what to do about moisture or water in the aid.

3. Presents a step-by-step program for getting used to the new hearing aid and for what to do about special adjustment problems encountered.

4. Outlines specific suggestions on what the speaker with normal hearing may do to make understanding easier for the hard-of-hearing listener, as well as directions for what the hard-of-hearing listener must do in order to improve his reception and perception of conversation.

5. Offers a different, step-by-step combined speech reading and auditory training approach and practice method. This does not rely on a frequently used technique of over-articulated whispering of unfamiliar material followed by hints, clues, and guesses until general comprehension is achieved. This method begins with total familiarity with the material on the part of the student. It concentrates on multiple visual and auditory stimulation, through a helper, followed by sight alone, sound alone, and combined sight-sound review. During this time the student is accumulating and storing visual and auditory images of speech sound, word, phrase, and sentence combinations which differ in each new context, depending on what preceded or what followed a given sound syllable, word, or sentence.

6. Gives, besides some conventional conversational phrase, sentence, and anecdote material, some unique combined vowel-consonant tables. These allow easy comparison of words by vowel differences and by high frequency consonant differences, either with sight or sound presentation. Furthermore, the method presents advanced and unique practice units which involve use of look-alike and sound-alike word pairs. Both words fit the meaning of the sentence, thus depriving the student of context cues and forcing him to learn subtle and little-used discrimination cues.

This is a workbook or manual of practical suggestions, directions, and lessons for the hard-of-hearing individual, to help him adjust better to his hearing aid, to take better care of the aid and to keep it operational, and to get the most out of it in terms of improved speech understanding. Furthermore, it presents a clinically proven and effective plan or method for combining speech reading and auditory training in one simple home practice procedure. Included are lesson materials, graded for difficulty from simple words and conversational phrases presented under ideal listening conditions up to complicated look-alike or sound-alike word pairs, both of which fit the context and which may be presented under difficult listening conditions.

INTRODUCTION

TO THE HEARING AID USER

IF you are a hard-of-hearing reader, you are to be commended. You have either just obtained a hearing aid, or are embarking on a home training program to develop skills in speech reading-auditory training, or both. You have realized that you have a hearing problem, accepted the fact, and are now seeking to do something about it. You are demonstrating your consideration for others near you who have been, or would be, inconvenienced by your failures in communication. In view of your interest in hearing improvement, this book has been prepared in order that you might find the adjustment and training easier and the wearing of a hearing aid more pleasant and helpful.

There are, of course, some things which may tend to discourage you. You must remember that a hearing aid does not restore hearing to normal. It only amplifies sound so that it is louder for you, and it sometimes improves the quality by various types of selective frequency emphases. If you place the whole burden of hearing restoration on your hearing aid, you will become dissatisfied in a short while. It is very important for you to recognize your responsibility in the training effort, which is to try your very best to adjust to the hearing aid and improve your speech understanding abilities.

If you have a mild loss, the chances are that you will make your adjustment in a short time. On the other hand, if your loss is more severe, your adjustment may well take quite a bit longer. Age is a factor in adjusting to a hearing aid. The elderly may find it difficult to change the listening habits of many years. Yet, it certainly can be done, as shown by the many senior citizens who have benefited in the past. The point to be made here is that you cannot expect to adjust to your hearing aid over night.

The success of your adjustment depends on you, your motivation for communication improvement, and your willingness to wear the aid regularly and consistently and to practice and work hard on the training.

It must be pointed out that there will be times of disappointment and perhaps embarrassment. This, however, happens in every phase of living. If you do become discouraged or self-conscious over your aid, remember the many prominent people who have worn hearing aids successfully in the past. Such outstanding persons as Winston Churchill and Bernard Baruch were among them. There are many famous men and women today, such as Nanette Fabray, Johnny Ray, and Norm Crosby, who not only wear their hearing aids consistently in public without embarrassment, but also talk freely about their benefit. They feel that a hearing aid is merely an aid to one of the senses that has become less keen, just as glasses are an aid to eyes that have become less keen. Wear your aid as nonchalantly as you do your glasses (if you wear them), and let it become a part of you. Your hearing aid is a sign that you are alert and outgoing and welcome the conversation of others.

Now let us begin the rehabilitation effort with a little basic background information. We will explain first, briefly, what the ear is like and how it works; then discuss types of hearing impairment and the kind of problems in communication that arise from them; and finally give a description of the degree and nature of your particular hearing problem, to be filled in by your audiologist or otologist.

THE NORMAL EAR AND HEARING FUNCTION

The ear is divided into three parts: an outer ear, a middle ear, and an inner ear. Sound waves pass along the canal of the outer ear and set the ear drum vibrating. Within the middle ear are three very small bones; the malleus, the incus, and the stapes. When the eardrum vibrates, these small bones are set into motion and transmit the sound vibrations across the middle ear to the inner ear. Within the inner ear is the organ for receiving sound. The sound vibrations which have passed through the outer ear are now transformed into nerve signals which are then sent to the brain for final recognition of sound.

TYPES OF HEARING IMPAIRMENT

If there is an impairment of the conduction of sound through either the external auditory canal or the middle ear, the type of hearing loss which results is known as *Conductive*. This impairment can usually be corrected or improved by medical treatment or surgery. The person with this loss does well with a hearing aid, because he needs only an increase in loudness of speech to make the sound clear.

If the site of the hearing impairment lies within the inner ear or in the nerve pathways to the brain, the type of hearing loss is called *Sensori-neural*. This type of impairment does not usually respond to medical or surgical treatment. The person with this type of loss may have slight to great difficulty with the clearness of words, even when they are very loud as when amplified by a hearing aid. The sound waves reach the inner ear but are not properly converted into an accurate message that can be passed on to the brain. For this person, it is very important to supplement what is heard with or without the hearing aid, with what is seen on the lips.

A person may have a combination of Conductive and Sensori-neural loss. Such a hearing impairment is known as a *Mixed Loss*.

YOUR HEARING PROBLEM

Based on your various hearing tests, your hearing problem can be generally summarized in the following chart.

Type of Loss	LEFT	RIGHT
(Conductive, Sensori-neural, Mixed)		
Average Decibel Loss		
(Units away from normal)		
Extent of Pure Tone Loss	NORMAL_____	NORMAL_____

in the Speech Range	MILD_____	MILD_____
	MODERATE_____	MODERATE_____
	MOD. SEVERE_____	MOD. SEVERE_____
	SEVERE_____	SEVERE_____
	PROFOUND_____	PROFOUND_____
Frequency Pattern of Greatest Loss		
	HIGH_____	HIGH_____
	FLAT_____	FLAT_____
	LOW_____	LOW_____
Extent of Speech Discrimination Loss	NORMAL_____	NORMAL_____
	MILD_____	MILD_____
	MODERATE_____	MODERATE_____
	MOD. SEVERE_____	MOD. SEVERE_____
	SEVERE_____	SEVERE_____
	PROFOUND_____	PROFOUND_____
Benefit with Best Hearing Aid (without speech reading)	EXCELLENT_____	EXCELLENT_____
	GOOD_____	GOOD_____
	FAIR_____	FAIR_____
	POOR_____	POOR_____
	NONE_____	NONE_____

REHABILITATIVE PROCEDURES

The first step in a rehabilitation program for your hearing problem is a complete examination by an ear, nose, and throat specialist (otolaryngologist). Usually at the same visit, your hearing is tested by an audiologist. The hearing test will reveal the amount and type of hearing loss and will assist the doctor in reaching a diagnosis and a decision as to treatment to be used. Sometimes a second visit to the audiologist may be necessary to permit further testing to aid in diagnosis of, and rehabilitation for, your problem.

The doctor will prescribe the appropriate treatment, which may be remedial or preventive, medical, or surgical.

When the otologist has established that no medical or surgical therapy is indicated, a hearing aid evaluation may be recommended by the audiologist, if the loss is of sufficient degree to warrant it. The hearing aid evaluation is a procedure designed to compare the test score performance of 6 to 8 instruments pre-selected by the audiologist as being most suitable for that patient's particular amplification needs. These amplification needs are established by carefully studying the original pure tone and speech earphone hearing test or audiogram. Such things will be noted as degree of sensitivity loss in each ear, quality of hearing as seen in the speech discrimination scores, shape of the pure tone threshold curves, and presence and degree of intolerance to loud sound. In addition, discussion with the patient will reveal how and where the aid will be used, and where on the body it probably should be worn. Many different types of instruments are available in the audiologist's trial library of aids (Fig. 1) which permit him to select models which can meet individual needs of high or low gain, high or low tone emphasis, limiting of total output for those with lowered tolerances, directional microphones, and place of wearing, either behind the ear, in glasses, on the body, or all-in-the-ear. In addition these specialized instruments will be

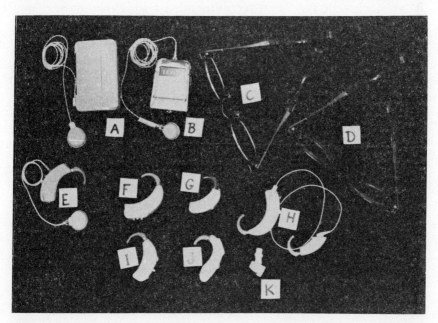

Figure 1. Types of Hearing Aids. (A) Power Body, (B) Regular Body, (C) Power CROS glasses, (D) Regular glasses, (E) Power Over-the-ear (OE) with external receiver, (F) Power OE, (G) Regular OE, (H) Power CROS OE, (I) Automatic Volume Control (AVC) OE, (J) Directional OE, (K) All-in-the-ear.

further modified by internal and external adjustments and alterations in the earpiece coupling system to be even more suitable for the patients needs. Each instrument will then be placed on the patient and his ability to hear faint speech and understand conversational speech established. The aid giving the most benefit will then be determined by test score comparison and a prescription given the patient for its purchase from a hearing aid dealer or it may be dispensed right there by some audiologists.

Nearly everyone with a hearing problem, not amenable to medical or surgical correction, should have the benefit of auditory rehabilitation. Such a program of rehabilitation may include all or some of the following: speech or lip reading, auditory training, guidance in using a hearing aid, speech conservation and improvement, and guidance in social adjustment. In your case, it has been recommended that you obtain:

1. _____Hearing Aid Evaluation
2. _____Guidance in Use of a Hearing Aid
3. _____Auditory Training
4. _____Speech Reading Lessons
5. _____Speech Improvement and Conservation
6. _____Guidance in Social Adjustment

Format of the Book

You will note that the book format contains chapters with similar titles and headings. This is because the chapters deal with the same skills of speech reading and auditory training, but in different levels of difficulty. The student should not proceed to higher levels of work in later chapters until the speech reader, helper, or the speech and hearing therapist is satisfied with the current progress.

CONTENTS

HELP FOR THE
HARD-OF-HEARING

— Chapter I —

INSTRUCTIONS FOR
HEARING AID USERS

FOR some time now, you have not been hearing sounds or speech as you used to. When you put on your hearing aid, you will be returning to a more natural world of sound. You will have to *train your ears* to accept these sounds again, and to make them meaningful. The young infant who is entering the world of hearing has a difficult adjustment to make in accepting and recognizing sounds; you have the advantage of having heard and recognized them before; you will merely need to get used to them again.

At first, it will seem to you that all of the noises in the world are conspiring to drown out the conversation of your friends and family and make you miserable. Airplane and bus motors, automobile horns, footsteps, cracking paper, and your own voice will all sound unnaturally loud to you with the aid. But remember, normal hearing people hear all of those sounds loudly too, but they have learned to ignore them — to push them subconsciously to the back of their minds — and to hear consciously only what they are listening for. You, too, can redevelop this ability by patient listening.

Even when you learn to disregard these "background noises," you may find that it is hard to understand all of the speech you hear or all of the sounds that are in your environment. This is a common complaint of new hearing aid users, but the difficulty can be overcome by determined practice and training.

The sound of your own voice will be too loud to you at first. This is due to two factors: You may have become accustomed to speaking louder than is necessary in order to be able to hear your own voice; and your own mouth will be closer than the other speaker's mouth to the microphone of your hearing aid. If you set the volume of the hearing aid to the most comfortable

3

level for your *own* voice, the speaker's voice will not be loud enough. You must adjust the volume control for the speaker's voice, and then lower the intensity of your own voice; you must gradually get used to it sounding "too loud." At first, your own voice, as well as other voices, may sound unnatural too, as anyone's voice does through an amplification system. Just as a loudspeaker, or recording system tends to "distort" one's voice to some degree, so the hearing aid produces some unnatural quality.

STEPS IN LEARNING TO USE A HEARING AID

The suggestions which follow are to use in training yourself for the most efficient use and quickest tolerance of your aid. You may adjust these suggestions to your needs and progress quickly or slowly to whatever degree suits you.

The First Few Days

Begin by wearing your aid indoors, in a quiet room. The aid should be worn a minimum of three times a day, approximately one hour each time. During these first few days, start with a low volume setting and gradually increase it. Do the following things:

1. Read aloud to yourself, to learn to adjust to your own voice. Speak clearly but naturally. Listen for the changing pitches. Do not speak *too* softly, as you must become used to hearing your own voice at a natural conversational level.
2. Talk with one person at a time, at no greater than a six-foot distance. Watch the speaker's lips attentively while listening. Ask him to speak in a clear, natural voice, not too fast nor too slow, and don't let him shout or "mouth" his words. In the evening, this can consist of a quiet "listening time" of five to ten minutes during which someone can read to you. By watching his lips all of the time, you can put together what you see and what you hear to make speech more meaningful. Watch for the differences on the

lips between sounds such as the "p" and "t," (as in pan and tan), the "b" and "y," (as in bet and yet), the "f" and "th" (as in fin and thin), and the "m" and "n" (as in met and net). (These are easily distinguished on the lips.)

3. Listen to environmental sounds. Try to identify car or airplane motors, clock ticking, footsteps, etc. Investigate each sound to discover its source.
4. Practice talking and listening to one person with a controlled sound background, such as a moderately loud radio or record player that plays music (to start with) and voices (later).
5. Begin to wear the hearing aid outdoors in reasonably quiet conditions.

During this time, note the times you practice. Keep notes on the words which are difficult for you to understand. Every night you may hand this list to whoever is assisting you, and have him make up a sentence with each word that you found difficult. He can then read the words of the sentence to you in a different order. Listen and watch carefully for clues, both auditory and visual, that will help you understand the words.

You should learn to relax while you are getting listening training. If you become tense or nervous while listening, you will not understand nearly as well. If you find yourself becoming too tense, turn off your aid (but leave it in your ear) and sit in an easy chair to relax for a few minutes.

The Next Week

Increase the time of wearing the aid to approximately two hours at a time, three times a day. Take care to rest if you tire easily or become nervous, but wear the aid as long as you can comfortably tolerate it. Arrange these listening situations in a quiet room.

1. Talk to several people at one time, at a distance of about six feet. Cross-conversation may be difficult at first, because you perhaps have lost the ability to catch the different voices. Pay attention to each speaker, watching his

lips while listening carefully to him. When he has stopped speaking, you can usually tell by the direction of his glance who is speaking next, and then you may shift your attention to the next speaker. Eventually you may even be able to follow a rapid-fire conversation at a bridge party. (But do not attempt this most difficult situation at first.)

2. Listen to the following things:

   a. You should have become accustomed to your aid so that you may begin listening to radio or TV commentators. Begin your aided watching or listening with programs which have very few speakers and little action in order to become accustomed to the differences between sound from the loudspeaker and sound originating in your own room. In order to avoid distortion of sound, you may wish to sit close to the loudspeaker at first with your volume turned low. Your goal should be comfortable hearing at about six feet. Gradually increase the volume setting up to at least a three-fourths level.

   b. Listen to various types of music over a radio, TV, or stereo. If your loss is greatest in the high pitches, listen especially for stringed instruments and sopranos. You may have difficulty with these sounds at first.

   c. While the vacuum cleaner is going or refrigerator is on, listen to someone talk. Relax and listen to the speech sounds and attempt to ignore the motor noise.

3. Keep up a "listening time" during which someone reads to you.

4. Constantly enlarge the list of words that are difficult for you. Have someone place these words in sentences as speech reading practice for you. Wear the hearing aid in all indoor situations.

The Next Few Weeks

Start to wear your instrument for a longer time, wherever you go, so that you will eventually be in the hearing world all day.

1. Go outside for a walk with the volume on your aid turned

very low. Listen carefully and identify all the sounds you hear, childrens voices, dogs barking, horns honking, etc. Do this every day alone until you are ready to have someone accompany you on your walk. Converse with this person and listen for his voice above the street noises.

2. Attend public meetings, beginning with church services or lectures. Sit as far front as possible, in the middle, in order to watch the lips of the speaker. Experiment with volume controls, to achieve the maximum hearing comfort. Later you can do the same thing in the movies. Avoid sitting under a balcony, as the sound will be distorted there. Best seating is found:

> At the movies: eight to fifteen rows from the front, and close to the center.
> At church and lectures: four to six rows from the front, and close to the center.

3. Listen to all types of radio and TV programs — music, news, plays. Always be relaxed but attentive.
4. Strive to have varied listening experiences both indoors and outdoors. Continue a "listening time" daily. By now you should be able to wear your aid most of the time.

It is best to find a uniform volume setting that you can use nearly all of the time, since the normal hearing person cannot turn his hearing up or down at a whim, and you are working toward normal hearing. However, you may wish to regulate your aid for extreme situations. On the street, you might want it turned fairly low, so that the background noises do not interfere with speech. At church or the theater, you may want to turn it fairly high to understand speech better.

You must remember there are many places where it may be difficult for you to understand speech. There are places where even the normal hearing individual has difficulty, such as very large rooms, churches, auditoriums, and theaters, all of which use amplification systems. You may also experience difficulty understanding speech in a noisy environment such as a cocktail party. People with normal hearing often have difficulty understanding under these listening conditions. Therefore, do not be discouraged if you cannot understand everything.

Follow this program closely until you have satisfied yourself and your family that you are getting maximum efficiency from your hearing aid. You may find that later you will become careless or lazy in your listening habits. If this happens start the training program over from the beginning until you have regained the lost ground.

CARE OF THE HEARING AID

1. Do not leave the aid in the sun or near a radiator, where it can be overheated. Also for the same reason, do not leave it in a closed car on a hot day.
2. Do not leave the aid where a dog can reach it. The plastics used in the hearing aids have certain characteristics which are appealing to dogs, causing aids to be frequently chewed up.
3. Do not drop (handle like a delicate electronic instrument).
4. Do not bend, twist, or snag the cord, if there is one.
5. Do not wear the aid when engaged in active play or sports where it could be struck, dislodged, or damaged.
6. Do not wear the hearing aid while applying hair spray.
7. Turn off the aid and open the battery compartment at night or when the aid is not in use.
8. Keep spare batteries on hand, and replace the batteries when the aid does not function or the power is weak.
9. Keep a spare cord on hand (if the aid uses a cord) and replace the cord when the sound starts to cut on and off.
10. If the hearing aid user is a child, the parents should listen to the hearing aid each morning to note humming, buzzing, static, or any other unusual sounds.
11. If you wear an ear level type of aid with earpiece and aid coupled with tubing, wipe off the earpiece periodically to clean it. Remove wax from the sound opening with a toothpick. It is better not to remove the earpiece from the tubing; let your hearing aid dealer or audiologist do that. If you wear a body type aid with external button receiver and snap-on earpiece, you should use the same method

for daily cleaning. Weekly you may snap the earpiece off the receiver and wash it in warm soapy water. Be sure to dry the sound opening afterwards. Do not snap the earpiece off too frequently as the receiver nubbin may become worn, making a loose coupling and feedback squeal. The replacement of a receiver is very expensive.

12. Several times a week do these things to reduce the build-up of corrosion, or whenever the aid does not work properly:

    a. Rub the battery ends with a rubber pencil eraser, rough cloth, or sole of a shoe.

    b. Rotate the volume control back and forth rapidly.

13. When putting in the battery or batteries, line up the + (plus) end of the battery with the + (plus) end of the battery compartment.

14. Each time the hearing aid is turned on, be sure that the earpiece is firmly seated in the ear and that the volume of the hearing aid is not on full gain, in order to prevent feedback squealing.

15. It is normal for the aid to squeal when not being worn in the ear, or when the volume is turned up.

    a. If squealing occurs frequently while the hearing aid is being worn, check the following:

       (1) See that the earpiece is firmly seated in the ear.

       (2) See that the volume has not been turned up to maximum.

       (3) See that the wearer is not seated in a corner or up close to a hard, reflecting surface.

       (4) See that the wearer's hand, cupped close to the hearing aid or to the ear when adjusting the hearing aid, is not the cause of the squealing.

    b. If the above have been checked and feedback squealing continues when the aid is worn, make the following tests:

       (1) Turn the hearing aid up to the normal comfortable setting and place your thumb tightly over the earpiece opening. If squealing is heard, there is a sound leak somewhere. You should have your

hearing aid dealer or audiologist check the aid.

(2) If no squealing occurs on the above test, by a process of elimination, the trouble lies in the earpiece, which is either too small or poorly fitted. See your dealer about a new, tighter fitting earpiece.

16. High humidity very frequently causes moisture to be deposited in the hearing aid amplifier components, the tubing, or the earpiece, leading to corrosion and intermittency of operation or reduction in power. The following suggestions will be helpful in this regard.
  a. Do not blow moisture out of your aid, receiver, tubing, or earpiece. This may only cause the deposit of additional moisture. Use a rubber bulb syringe to blow it out.
  b. Use a silica gel-air dryer in a plastic bag or a box to put the aid in at night to absorb all the moisture. Get it from your hearing aid dealer.
17. Some occupations and hobbies requiring vigorous exercise outdoors in the sun or indoors in high temperature surroundings, cause heavy perspiration which may interfere with proper hearing reception or eventually cause damage to the instrument. These suggestions will help:
  a. Wear an elastic sweatband around your head.
  b. Using a roll-on antiperspirant, rub some on your little finger. Then rub this material in the outer ear canal.
  c. Roll on some more antiperspirant behind your ear.
  d. From a rubber corn pad or corn plaster cut out a rubber insulator to be stuck to the inside surface of the aid normally in contact with the mastoid area.
  e. Put your aid in the silica-gel air dryer sack each night.
18. Should the instrument be immersed in water, or take on large quantities of water, do these things:
  a. Sling out the water by vigorous shaking.
  b. Blot up any water with blotter or absorbent paper.
  c. Wrap the aid in absorbent paper.
  d. Bring or send the aid in to your hearing aid dealer as soon as possible.

19. To get the hearing aid on and in place in the ear, do the following things:

   a. Take hold of the outer ear in the back and pull it outwards and downwards with one hand.

   b. With the other hand, guide the top of the earpiece into the notch or groove above the canal.

   c. Push the earpiece canal tip part into the ear canal and the large rounded part of the earpiece down into the hollows of the ear until it slips into place and becomes "part of the ear" and feels comfortable and tight. You may find that certain ears may require an alternative method to replace steps "b" and "c." Start the canal portion of the earpiece into the ear canal with the helix tip part pointing toward the eye, then rotate the earpiece backwards until the tip slips into the helical groove.

Chapter II

SPEECH READING AND AUDITORY TRAINING PROGRAM

Purpose

THE purpose of this series of speech reading and auditory training lessons is to help you *begin* to achieve your maximum ability for understanding speech.

WHAT IS SPEECH READING?

More and more frequently the term "speech reading" is being used instead of the older designation "lip reading" because it is important to stress the idea that the entire face and neck area (not just the lips) must be observed by the hard-of-hearing listener and viewer for cues to understand what is being said by the speaker.

Another reason for using the term "speech reading" is that many people resist embarking on this type of training when designated "lip reading" as there seems to be some sort of stigma attached to its use. As a matter of fact many hard-of-hearing people, when asked, will vigorously deny ever having used lip reading as though it were something offensive or shameful. Actually silent movie comprehensive tests with normal hearing students have shown that even they speech (lip) read without realizing it and the hard of hearing do even more, whether or not they have had instruction.

When lip reading training is recommended, many hard-of-hearing people respond by saying "I'm not *that* deaf, surely." Far too few people realize that any hard-of-hearing person may benefit from speech reading no matter how severe or mild their loss. Usually it is even more important for the person with a loss too mild for a hearing aid, but with speech understanding and communication problems, to get lip reading instruction, than it is for the person with a more severe loss who may be compensating better by using a hearing aid.

Another misconception that people have which makes them resistant to lip reading training, is that the speaker will be self-conscious and uncomfortable if the hard-of-hearing person looks at his mouth as he speaks. At normal conversational distance, the speaker cannot tell if the listener is looking at his mouth, chin, nose, or eyes. So the lip-reader can look intently at the speaker's face, concentrating his main focus on the lips and mouth without fear of bothering the speaker at all. As a matter of fact he will be flattered at the indication of interest and attention shown to his words.

Still another reason people give for not using lip reading is that sometimes circumstances make it difficult or impossible to lip-read well, as for instance when light conditions are very poor, or if the speaker's back is turned, his face or mouth are temporarily covered, or he mumbles with little or no lip movement. However, to totally reject the concept or attempt the use of lip reading for these reasons is like refusing ever to eat because sometimes cooking facilities are primitive, or only poor cooks are available for the food preparation. We must do the best we can under difficult listening or lip reading circumstances, and certainly use lip reading as much as we possibly can when conditions are satisfactory.

Speech reading is understanding what is being said by watching the speaker's face — *in particular the movements of the lips.* For those with hearing problems, speech reading is a means by which they can keep up with a conversation which is either only partly heard or not heard at all. A listener, while keeping his eyes on a speaker's face, subconsciously forms an association between the sounds of speech and the corresponding movements of the mouth. Not all sounds can be seen and understood by looking alone. However, our minds will fill in the missing parts of a sentence so that it is not essential to try to understand every sound or word a speaker utters in conversation.

WHAT IS AUDITORY TRAINING?

Auditory training is educating an individual with a hearing loss to make as much use as possible of the hearing which he does have and to make his listening more efficient. It involves teaching a person, through listening practice, to make meaning out of imperfect, distorted sound. Such learning may be undertaken whether the individual wears a hearing aid or not.

SPEECH READING AND AUDITORY TRAINING COMBINED

The great majority of hard-of-hearing people gain the best result by combining speech reading and auditory training. Studies have shown that when speech reading and hearing are combined, better results are obtained than when speech reading or hearing are used independently of each other. For example, auditory training will help the individual to recognize those sounds which are difficult to see, or to distinguish words that look alike, while speech reading helps a person to recognize those sounds which may be difficult to hear, or to distinguish words which sound alike. Eventually by combining speech reading and auditory training, an individual may not be aware of just how much he is getting from speech reading and how much he is actually hearing. If you have a hearing aid you should wear the aid during all practice sessions. As you progress in speech reading, you should practice under more difficult circumstances, such as having the speaker speak to you either from the side, or moving his head, or partly obscuring his lips. Speech reading at this stage should also be given at different distances, starting off close to the speaker and gradually moving farther away. Remember, there is no end point when you have completed your speech reading training. It is like learning to play the piano. The longer you practice, the better or more skilled you become.

SPEECH READING AND AUDITORY
TRAINING INSTRUCTIONS

There are *three important rules* to follow as you use your

speech reading and auditory training in conversation.

1. Concentrate the attention on the thought that is being expressed rather than on individual words. This is the way anyone understands when he hears, or when he reads the printed page.
2. Do not interrupt a speaker before he has finished a sentence to ask him to repeat what he said. The speech-reader will often find that although he does not understand the first part of a sentence, he does understand the last part. In many cases, this gives him the thought of the whole sentence, without repetition by the speaker being necessary.
3. Form the habit of watching the speaker's lips at all times, even when hearing without difficulty. Then, if the speaker's voice drops, the speech-reader who has formed this habit, is in a position to go on understanding by means of speech reading, sometimes without being conscious of the fact that the voice has dropped. Do not be reluctant to fix your gaze directly on the speaker's mouth. Do not be concerned that by so doing, the speaker will become self-conscious. As stated before, at normal conversational distances, he will not be able to tell if you are looking at his mouth, nose, chin, or eyes. Remember, do not use as an excuse for not watching the speaker's lips, that many speakers mumble and provide few lip cues, or that sometimes the lighting is poor and you cannot see the lips well. This in no way alters the fact that whenever you *can* watch the speaker's mouth, your speech understanding will be enhanced. Some lip reading is better than no lip reading at all.

The following instructions are designed to help you understand speech to the best of your ability.

TO THE HARD-OF-HEARING LISTENER

It is very common to have a type of hearing loss which permits you to *hear* the spoken voice but at the same time does not allow you to get the words clear. Do not assume that everyone else, in speaking to you, is mumbling, or that they have "mush in their mouths." Recognize that if you often "hear but have trouble getting the words clear" or "speech runs together," that the trouble is not with the speaker, but in *your* ears. You will need to fill in the gaps by learning to speech read, either by taking lessons from a teacher, or practicing at home. The following will also help you to be a better speech-reader.

If you are a hard-or-hearing person with speech under-standing problems you *must* do the following things in conversation:

1. Pay very close attention with your eyes and ears to the speaker.
2. Keep a lively interest in conversation even when listening and speech reading conditions are difficult.
3. Have confidence in your listening-speech reading ability. Do not give up when the going gets tough.
4. On the other hand, do not be overconfident. Do not fake or pretend understanding. Ask for clarification of a missed thought or idea rather than repetition of each word.
5. Focus your gaze on the speaker's face at all times, especially the mouth.
6. Adjust your position so that you have the best light possible on the speaker's face, not on yours.
7. Keep up, always, with the current word being said. Do not get bogged down on one difficult word or phrase. If you keep up, repetition and context will fill the gaps.
8. Look and listen for key words and phrases. Each small individual word need not be identified.

TO THE NORMAL HEARING SPEAKER

For some people, hearing speech in conversation is like listening to a radio with a broken speaker. The voice may be loud enough but the words are fuzzy and run together, and cannot be clearly separated or understood. They understand some words and some voices better than others depending on the pitch range and on how much speech reading they can do. It is often said that these people "hear when they want to hear," but this is not true. It also should be stressed that their misunderstanding of spoken words is no reflection on their intelligence. The trouble lies in a defect in their hearing mechanism.

In order that the speaker can be better understood in conversation, the speaker should follow these rules in conversation:

1. *Do not shout,* especially do not shout if the listener wears a hearing aid.
2. Look directly at the listener, (speech reader).
3. Do not cover your mouth with books, newspapers or hands.
4. Do not speak with cigar, cigarette, or pipe in your mouth.
5. Hold your head still and steady when speaking.
6. Adjust your position so the light (from lamp or window) is on your face, not on the speech-reader's face.
7. Get in close enough to allow easy observation of your face (within six feet) but not so close that easy observation of the whole face is difficult, or so that the listener — lip reader is uncomfortable by your nearness (usually no closer than two feet).
8. Speak slowly — but not unnaturally.
9. Speak distinctly, but naturally; do not slur, mumble, or mouth your words.
10. If the listener fails to get your meaning, rephrase or re-word, rather than repeat. It is more effective and less embarrassing to the listener who is hard-of-hearing.
11. Be considerate and patient.

VOICES — YOUR OWN AND OTHER PEOPLE'S

What do other people say about your voice when you wear your aid? Do they say it is still too loud? Do they say it is too soft? Does it sound like your voice is too loud to you? Here are some explanations for your observations:

1. If you wear an aid, your mouth is closer to the micro-

phone than the speaker's mouth, therefore making your voice more amplified and louder.

2. Your own voice was too loud before you wore an aid to compensate for your hearing loss, and now this speaking habit remains.

3. You are accustomed to a world of soft sounds before you wore an aid. Now even normal sounds seem too loud.

4. You may have a very common problem associated with nerve type hearing losses — that of unusually rapid growth in loudness. This means you require amplification in order for sound to be heard, but slightly higher levels suddenly become loud or too loud. It is to be hoped that part of this problem has been taken care of by a specially designed output limiting feature of your hearing aid. The rest must be taken care of by gradual adjustment through time, practice, and experience. If poor tolerance of sound persists beyond a few months, consult with your audiologist or rehabilitation therapist.

Do not overcompensate for your voice being loud, by turning the volume of your aid down too low to permit your best understanding, or by lowering your voice level until it is difficult to be heard by others. Rather, keep your voice at a level considered normal by your listeners, recognizing that eventually it will be normal for you also.

NOISES AND SOUNDS AROUND YOU

Identification, recognition, and discrimination of noise and sounds must precede a more subtle identification, recognition, and discrimination of words and combinations of words in conversational speech.

Whenever sounds are new, different, or unidentified, investigate immediately by seeking sources and/or inquiring as to their origin. Check off the sounds as you now begin to notice them:

1. Noises around the house (telephone, doorbell, clocks, watches, vacuum, washer, drier)

2. Musical instruments
3. Sports and recreation
4. Tools and machines
5. Animals, birds, and insects
6. Transportation (trains, airplanes, approaching cars)
7. Food preparation
8. Heating and cooling (air conditioner, fan or blower, re-frigerator)
9. Water running
10. Weather
11. Records and radio
12. Live voices

Are you beginning to discriminate the general noises and sounds as noted in previous paragraphs and your own particular household noises and sounds?
List sounds you have recently identified:

List sounds you are still having trouble noticing:

Just as gross sounds and noises in the environment must be gradually identified, recognized, and discriminated, speech sounds which are much more complex and involve more subtle sound differences, must also be gradually identified, recognized, and discriminated.
Here are some words you may have difficulty understanding:

WORDS	SENTENCES
wonderful	We had a *wonderful* time at the party.
television	The *television* program lasted for two hours.
serious	The man had a *serious* look on his face.
envelope	Enclosed in the letter was a self-addressed, stamped *envelope*.

WORDS	*SENTENCES*
animals	We looked at all the different *animals* at the pet store.
different	My father has many *different* hats.
drawer	We keep the scissors in the *drawer*.
violence	There's a lot of *violence* on TV.
watching	We were *watching* them play the game.
particular	She is very *particular* about her hair.
family	There are seven children in his *family*.
children	My *children* were making too much noise.
elbow	I bumped my *elbow* on the table
discouraged	He became *discouraged* after the first day.
president	The *President* made a speech on television.

List below your own sentences containing words you have found to be difficult.

SUMMARY

1. The diagnosis and treatment of your hearing problem should occur only after otological examination and audiologic testing.

2. If your hearing can be improved through medication or surgery, your doctor will tell you. If not, a training program should be started.

3. If a hearing aid is prescribed, you should purchase it as soon as possible. Usually some form of training should follow the purchase to help you adjust to the aid and also to get the maximum benefit from it.

4. Speech reading combined with auditory training brings about the best result for the understanding of speech. The success of speech reading depends upon your interest and determination to improve.

5. When practicing speech reading, try to remain relaxed.

6. Try to place the speaker in favorable lighting conditions, preferably with the light falling on his face, not on yours. Shadows on his face, or light in your eyes will make your task more difficult. The maximum distance you should be from a speaker should be six feet, and the minimum should be about two feet.

7. Do not try to get every word in a conversation. Rather go for the general meaning. Key words will appear which will help you do this.

8. Do not try to hide your hearing loss or attempt to control and monopolize the conversation. Remember, if you have not understood, tell the speaker so that when he gets to the end of a sentence, he may repeat or rephrase the sentence.

9. Keep a constant check on your own voice and speech. Do not shout or whisper.

10. It is your responsibility to train those around you to speak in a manner which will give you maximum understanding.

11. Constant practice and patience is required on your part; and the success of a training program depends upon your cooperativeness, attitude, and acceptance of the problem.

Chapter III

GENERAL PROCEDURE FOR
SPEECH READING PRACTICE

YOU are now ready to start a formal approach to speech reading and auditory training to help you understand speech better. Do not make the mistake of thinking that simultaneous speech reading and auditory listening are incompatible — that one detracts or prevents you from doing well with the other. Speech reading and auditory discrimination go hand-in-hand, complementing each other.

GROUP I SENTENCES

We begin by giving you a key word in the sentence. These key words are written to the left of the sentence on the practice sheets, for example;

bought — We bought a house.

Your helper should show you the sentence or phrase for you to read aloud, so you will know what it is, and then say the key word so you can both see and hear it. He should then say the sentence so you can both see and hear it also. You should repeat the sentence back to him so he knows you have the meaning. Then he says the sentence hiding his lips, so you hear it without speech reading help. Following this, he repeats the sentence using *no* voice so you can watch the movement of his lips. Finally, he should speak the sentence allowing you to both speech read and hear the sentence. You should then repeat the sentence back to him. Each sentence on the practice sheets should be done following the above procedure.

SUMMARY OF THE PROCEDURE

1. Helper shows you the phrase or sentence for you to read aloud.

2. Helper says the key word and then the sentence containing the key word. You should watch and listen, then repeat the sentence. If you do not understand the sentence, the helper will repeat it.
3. Helper says the sentence hiding his lips and you will listen.
4. Helper says the sentence without using his voice and you watch.
5. Helper repeats the sentence naturally while you watch and listen.
6. You should now repeat the sentence back to your helper.

After all of the sentences have been completed, the helper may choose any of the sentences to give you (after first telling you the key word).

The method, described above, does not limit practice drill to guessing for general meaning of the material. You practice, knowing what is going to be seen and heard. This allows you to concentrate all your attention on fixing or remembering what all the speech sound combinations look like and sound like, so that you can use this knowledge for better understanding of conversation. By concentrating your total attentional powers on how these particular word combinations look and how they sound, you begin to memorize and store these experiences for future use. These many listening and watching repetitions of known material are essential because words and phrases as well as sounds look different, depending on what sounds and words precede and what sounds and words follow a given word.

GROUP II SENTENCES

These are medium difficulty sentences. The key word is not shown first, as was done in Group I. Proceed as for Group I sentences and begin Step 2 of the above procedure.

GROUP III SENTENCES

These are the hardest sentences. They are based on the same

topic. They are arranged in pairs with the second sentence of each pair being a continuation of the thought of the first sentence. Give the first sentence of the pair, and wait for the speech-reader to say the sentence back to you. Then give the associated sentence. When all the sentences have been repeated correctly by the speech-reader, go back over the whole group, giving both sentences of each pair without pausing between them. Then again use the steps for speech reading training as were outlined previously, starting now at Step 3.

HOW TO USE THE CONVERSATIONAL DRILLS

The speech reader should read the title out loud, and then the helper should give the first sentence. When this has been understood, conversational variations of this sentence should be attempted. Then read the next sentence, and proceed as above. Finally review all the sentences out of order. Encourage the speech-reader to make his own responses to the sentences. In this way a more natural conversational speech reading lesson is obtained.

CONVERSATIONAL PRACTICE

During this period of training, have a five to ten minute conversation speech reading practice, based on an article you and your helper have read in a newspaper or magazine. During this practice try to obtain the general meaning of the conversation, rather than speech read every word. If you should become tense or tired, stop and relax, before attempting to do more speech reading. Do not interrupt the speaker until he has finished his sentence, as you will discover the meaning of what he is saying as he continues speaking. We all tend to repeat ourselves or to rephrase; if you do not understand something the first time, chances are you will pick it up on the next go-round. That is, if you do not let yourself get hung up on one word, building your frustration and distracting yourself from the subsequent speech. Always try to keep up with the current words being said, and to forget those parts missed.

During this period keep a list of difficult words encountered in conversation. Have your helper write these in sentences. Then using these words as key words, practice the sentences as outlined in the steps for speech reading.

INSTRUCTIONS FOR THE HELPER

When you are giving the lessons, do the following things:

1. Speak at a normal speech rate.
2. Speak with natural intonations of your voice.
3. Do not stop until you have said a whole sentence.
4. Do not speak too slowly, or too rapidly.
5. Form the words clearly with an active mouth but do not mouth your words or use exaggerated lip movements.
6. If the speech-reader fails to understand:
   a. Repeat the whole sentence, exactly as it is written.
   b. If he still does not understand, write a key word to help give him the meaning, and repeat the sentence again.
   c. If he still does not understand, show the sentence and then repeat the sentence for him.
7. When practicing the conversational drills, read them silently first and then say them naturally, the way you would in normal conversation. Example sentence: "Do you think it will rain?" you should say it, "D'ya think it'll rain?"

When you are talking with the speech reader in *normal conversation:*

1. Do suggestions 1 through 5 above.
2. Keep your head still.
3. Do not hide your lips with your hands, glasses, cigarettes, books or newspapers.
4. If the speech reader fails to understand, do not repeat over and over. It is much better for you to reword or rephrase the sentence in a different way.

By now, you should be starting to get used to your aid. The suggestions from Chapter I should be continued to help you fully adjust to your aid. Keep reading aloud to yourself for five minutes. Gradually you will find that the sound of your voice will become more natural. Also, make special note of the voices of someone you hear every day such as your wife or husband and note if her or his voice is also becoming more natural to you. Make a point of watching and listening to the TV news each day and listen to the quality of the newscaster's voice.

Reread the section in Chapter I, concerning care of your aid. Make sure you are carrying out the instructions, so that you get the best use from your instrument. Make remarks at the end of this Chapter, under the heading, *Hearing Aid Adjustment,* concerning your reactions to the aid. Especially note if sounds such as the phone or cars, etc. are becoming more natural.

Remember, in conversation do not try to understand every word said to you. Instead, listen for the general meaning of the sentence. However, in your speech reading practice drill it is necessary to not only understand each and every word, but to note and remember how each sound and word looks and sounds in different combinations depending on what precedes or follows the given sound, syllable, word, or sentence.

Group I Sentences

1. *went*   I went shopping.
We went to the store.
She went for a ride.

2. *stores*   The stores were very crowded.
All the stores had Christmas decorations.
It was very noisy in the stores.

3. *bought*   I bought some presents.
I also bought some milk.
Have you bought your presents yet?

4. *TV*   I went shopping for a new TV set.
The color TV sets were expensive.
Do you have a color TV set?

5. *toy*   The toy department was full of children.
The toy cars were very popular.
All the kids liked to drive the toy cars.

6. *presents* Presents are getting more expensive.
It seems impossible to buy a present under $5.00.
I paid $30.00 for two presents.

7. *windows* The store windows were all decorated.
Some of the windows were very beautiful.
The men were cleaning the windows.

Group II Sentences

1. It was difficult to park the car.
   The parking lot was full of cars.
   There were a lot of cars on the freeway.

2. Most of the children were riding bicycles.
   The children got out of school one hour early.
   Tell the children not to make so much noise.

3. We don't have enough room in this apartment.
   There's too much furniture in this room.
   There's a lot of room in the backyard.

4. Ride your bicycle to the store.
   My bicycle has a flat tire.
   He's not allowed to take his bicycle to school.

5. Our newspaper got wet in the rain.
   We stopped at the store to pick up a newspaper.
   Our dog chewed up the newspaper.

6. We played our new records.
   The old records were scratched.
   They kept the records in a metal box.

7. They have a very strange looking dog.
   The drink tasted very strange.
   The shoes that she had looked strange.

8. It was very exciting to see you working again.
   The exciting movie stimulated the audience.
   The final game of the season was exciting.

9. He was a very successful businessman.
   I hope I can be as successful as you have been.
   Our baseball team was very successful that year.

10. My sister is a very creative person.
    My mother writes with a creative flair.
    The creative flower arrangement was expensive.

11. I went shopping because I needed some new clothes.
    Stop talking, because the loud noise bothers me!
    She left work because she felt ill.

12. The entrance will be blocked at eight o'clock.
    Don't forget to slow down before you come to the entrance.
    Why do people always exit through the entrance?

13. My education should help me to get a good job.
    My mother always told me that education was important.
    My teacher always told me that she was preparing me for
    higher education.

14. My hearing loss has caused me to watch people's lips at all
    times.
    I feel like I am hearing noises all the time.
    The hearing has been set for Monday at ten o'clock.

Group III Sentences

1. It was very exciting to see you working again.
   I hope you take it easy at first, and don't over do it.

2. He was a very successful businessman.
   Everyone in town seemed to like and respect him.

3. My sister is a very creative person.
   She has developed her skills in painting and sculpture.

4. I went shopping because I needed some new clothes.
   All my old clothes are too short and out of date.

5. The entrance will be blocked at eight o'clock.
   We will begin the ballgame as soon as possible.

6. My education should help me to get a good job.
   It will be my responsibility to show that I can do the job.

7. My hearing loss has caused me to watch people's lips at all times.
   My understanding of speech has improved a great deal.

ONE WORD SENTENCE CONVERSATIONAL DRILL

1. Hi
2. Ouch
3. Fantastic
4. Great
5. Wow
6. Wonderful
7. Terrific
8. Grand
9. Unbelievable
10. Sorry
11. Quiet
12. Super
13. Gee
14. Magnificent
15. Courageous
16. Stop
17. Shocking
18. Bravo
19. Exit
20. Yield

PHRASE CONVERSATIONAL DRILL

1. Keep out
2. Keep off the grass
3. No smoking
4. Beward of dog
5. No hunting allowed
6. Stop for school bus
7. Quiet hospital zone
8. Do not enter
9. One way only
10. Stop for pedestrians
11. Walk, don't run
12. No drinks or food allowed
13. Do not handle merchandise
14. Employees only
15. No swimming in this area
16. No loitering
17. Slow down for signal ahead
18. Watch out for falling rocks
19. Slippery when wet
20. Private property—Keep out

21. Narrow bridge
22. Free samples—Take one
23. No minors allowed
24. School zone—Slow down
25. No soliciting
26. Traffic signal ahead
27. Curves ahead
28. Detour ahead
29. Adults only
30. Men at work
31. Construction ahead
32. Members only
33. No talking
34. Do not litter
35. Railroad crossing
36. Wet paint
37. Loose gravel
38. Off limits
39. Caution
40. No alcoholic beverages

PHRASE CONVERSATIONAL DRILL

About Weather

1. Partly cloudy
2. Fifty percent chance of rain
3. Hot and dry
4. Warning — Tornado Watch
5. Misty and damp
6. Snow flurries
7. Icy roads
8. Gusty winds
9. Ten below zero
10. Warm and sunny
11. Possible thunder showers
12. Flood warnings
13. Light showers
14. Hurricane warning

SENTENCE CONVERSATIONAL DRILL

When You Meet

1. How are you?
2. It's nice to meet you.
3. I haven't seen you for ages.
4. Where have you been?
5. How's your family?
6. How've you been?
7. I saw your brother yesterday.
8. Come over and see us.
9. We've moved to a new house.
10. My phone number is 271-4231.
11. Call us up. We're home most of the time.
12. Give my regards to Barbara.
13. I must go now.
14. It was good seeing you.
15. Goodbye. Glad I met you.

SENTENCE CONVERSATIONAL DRILL

At the Dinner Table

1. Pass the salt, please.
2. This meatloaf looks very good.
3. May I have some more gravy?
4. These potatoes are delicious.
5. I would like wine with my dinner.
6. I don't care for any water, thank you.
7. This steak is very tender.
8. I may be too full to eat dessert.
9. May I have another glass of milk?
10. I will help with the dinner dishes.
11. Would you rather wash or dry?
12. Do you have enough for a second helping?
13. The vegetables were fresh and crisp.
14. I would like some dressing for my salad.
15. Let's go for a walk when we are finished.

SENTENCE CONVERSATIONAL DRILL

High Cost of Living

1. The cost of living has gone up tremendously in the last few years.
2. It seems as though food prices go up every day.
3. Our rent was raised $35.00 last month.
4. Our utilities are unbelievably high.
5. To lower our gasoline bill we bought an economy car.
6. Last week my boss gave me a cost of living raise.
7. Last month I had to pay my income taxes.
8. I hope we are able to save enough for a summer vacation.
9. The President promised to lower our taxes.
10. The interest rate on the loan was very high.
11. We paid $35.00 for our telephone bill last month.
12. We had to borrow $700.00 from the bank.
13. I hope the new administration can lower the high cost of living.
14. Gasoline prices are expected to increase.
15. Inflation seems to affect everyone.

Hearing Aid Adjustment

Note your reaction to your aid. What improvement in hearing have you noticed? Do your own and others' voices sound more natural? Are there still some difficulties? Note these difficulties on this page.

Chapter IV

COMBINING AUDITORY TRAINING
AND SPEECH READING

VOICE ATTRIBUTES

EACH day have a ten-minute listening period while someone reads to you. Have the person read to you using different degrees of loudness. Sometimes the reader's voice should be soft, sometimes loud, and at other times normal. Make a note on your practice sheet of which level of loudness is easiest for you to understand.

During the week, have special practice periods in which you listen to the voices of people who are speaking to you. In particular, take notice of the following three attributes of voice:

PITCH

LOUDNESS

QUALITY

For pitch and loudness, note if the person's voice is high, average, or low. For quality, note if the voice is harsh, breathy, husky, shrill, or normal, etc. Use your own words to describe the voice and make a daily note on the practice sheet of at least one person's voice you have analyzed.

Again this week, listen to environmental noises. However, this time begin to analyze them, using the three qualities of sound mentioned above.

PITCH

LOUDNESS

QUALITY

By now you should be wearing your aid full time, (see Chapter I) and you should gradually be getting more adjusted to it. If noises (such as those of the street) still seem abnormally loud to you, turn the gain control down slightly. Remember,

39

however, that you will gradually become more and more accustomed to such loud noises and eventually you will not have to alter the setting of the hearing aid. Make sure you are completely familiar with the instructions on "Care of Your Aid" from Chapter I, and that you are carrying out these instructions regularly.

HOW TO USE STORIES FOR LISTENING AND SPEECH READING PRACTICE

In Chapter IV, we begin the use of stories for practice drill. The following procedure is recommended for listening and speech reading practice. This lesson material, like the phrase and sentence drills, will require a helper.

The speech-reader should read the title of the story. Proper names should be shown and said to the speech-reader. The helper should read the story aloud, allowing the speech-reader to interrupt at the end of a sentence if he has not understood the meaning. Then the helper should read the story again. Again the speech-reader should attempt to follow the meaning, only stopping the helper when there is a pause at the end of a sentence.

If the speech-reader has followed the general meaning, but has missed many words as the story is read, it should be read again. The speech-reader should now indicate if he misses important words, so that they may be repeated. The helper should then ask questions about the story, and have the speech-reader answer them.

You should now be combining auditory training with speech reading to help you understand the speech of others. Keep up a daily conversation practice, using a TV program or an article from a paper as a point of discussion. Remember to follow the general rules outlined in Chapter I.

Group I Sentences

1. *breakfast*   Breakfast is ready.
Do you want coffee with your breakfast?
Let's wash the breakfast dishes.

2. *corn flakes* Do you like corn flakes?
Pour milk over your corn flakes.
Corn flakes with bananas taste good.

3. *orange*   Pour the orange juice.
A small glass of orange juice will do.
Put the orange juice in the refrigerator.

4. *bacon*   I had bacon and eggs for breakfast.
Put the bacon in the pan.
This is good bacon.

7. *lunch*   It's lunch time.
I ate a sandwich for lunch.
How long do you get for lunch?

6. *milk*   Do you want a glass of milk?
The milk is in the pitcher.
Don't spill the milk on the table.

7. *supper*   What time do you eat supper?
I enjoy eating supper out.
Did you say that supper was ready?

Group II Sentences

1. The flowers had a lovely fragrance.
   Stop on the side of the road and pick some flowers.
   Don't let the dog dig in the flowers.

2. Put a cover on the couch.
   The couch was as comfortable as a bed.
   A drink was spilled on the couch last night.

3. Don't follow me when I leave.
   You go ahead and I will follow.
   That little dog will follow you anywhere.

4. The candle shop smelled good.
   The smell from the candle shop was pleasant.
   Our candles were burning all night.

5. The doorbell woke me up.
   I wonder if the doorbell is working?
   The doorbell sounds like chimes.

6. I will hang all the pictures tonight.
   Let's go to the gallery and pick up a new picture.
   I can't picture you as a football player.

7. The woman went all over town to find the right purse.
   She can put everything in that purse.
   I am going to get that purse for my wife.

8. The department store will be closed Sunday.
   Our department carries all different brands.
   This department seems to get all of the hard jobs.

9. Everyone seems happy whenever you come to sing.
   I'll stop everyone from making so much noise.
   This job will have enough work for everyone.

10. This dedication will be rewarded.
    I have never seen so much dedication in one department.
    Dedication and hard work are necessary traits.

11. I'll have a hamburger without onions.
    I want four hamburgers to go.
    Could we have hamburgers today instead of hotdogs?

12. I am wearing my new clothes tomorrow for church.
    Please, do not wear those shoes when you go out to play.
    Could I wear my new tennis shoes at the picnic?

13. We are all members of the same team.
    The members of the club will meet here tomorrow for dinner.
    Our club has many loyal members.

14. I hope this problem won't come between us.
    There is a disagreement between the manager and the workers.
    I could not decide between getting new shoes or a new shirt.

Group III Sentences

1. The department store will be closed on Sunday.
   It will open again at nine o'clock on Monday morning.

2. Everyone seems happy whenever you come to sing.
   Your voice has a quiet and tender quality.

3. This dedication will be rewarded.
   Your loyalty and enthusiasm will help us succeed.

4. I'll have a hamburger without onions.
   Could you put my order in a sack to go?

5. I am wearing my new clothes tomorrow for church.
   It will be my first chance to wear them.

6. We are all members of the same team.
   We should all work together so we can win the championship.

7. I hope this problem won't come between us.
   We should be able to work well together.

PHRASE CONVERSATIONAL DRILL

Descriptive Language

1. Beautiful picture
2. Breathtaking view
3. Shiny car
4. Silky hair
5. Plush carpet
6. Rough wood
7. Super job
8. Great catch
9. Good hit
10. Fine run
11. Good pitch
12. Slender hands
13. Golden tan
14. Sweet smelling hands
15. Interesting book
16. Soft material
17. Tropical plant
18. Fluffy clouds
19. Clear sky
20. Spicy tea

PHRASE CONVERSATIONAL DRILL

About Work

1. All employees must punch in
2. Coffee break
3. Take a letter
4. Have a seat
5. Out to lunch
6. Fill in the blanks
7. File all copies
8. Dictation box
9. Bring these charts to me
10. Label all folders
11. Are you finished with your work
12. Employees only
13. Office memo
14. Return all calls
15. Closed on Labor Day

SENTENCE CONVERSATIONAL DRILL

About the Weather

1. It sure is humid today.
2. Do you think it'll rain?
3. I'd better wear a coat.
4. Is it raining yet?
5. This is the worst rain I've ever seen.
6. Did you bring an umbrella?
7. I left my umbrella at home.
8. Is it hot enough for you today?
9. This is the hottest summer we've had in years.
10. It's very warm, so you won't need a coat.
11. I think it'll be cooler tonight.
12. Fall is my favorite time of the year.
13. Let's go for a ride and see the autumn leaves.
14. Did you get any frost last night?
15. We had to cover our shrubs to keep 'em from freezing.

SENTENCE CONVERSATIONAL DRILL

Time

1. What time is it?
2. Do you have the time?
3. Is it time to go yet?
4. What time does the show start?
5. If we don't hurry we'll be late.
6. What time does the bus get in?
7. The train is running late.
8. What time does your plane leave?
9. I haven't time to do that now.
10. The show starts at eight o'clock.
11. You have an appointment at 4:30 PM on Wednesday.
12. It took me an hour to drive home.
13. What time are you leaving?
14. The clock is fast.
15. We'll be there at six o'clock.

SENTENCE CONVERSATIONAL DRILL

When Shopping for Clothes

1. Would you like to go to the shopping center with me?
2. I need to buy some new clothes.
3. This is a huge department store.
4. Where is the dress department?
5. They have a large selection of blouses.
6. I think a size 9 will fit.
7. They have many nice ties.
8. I could not find the right color shirt.
9. He wanted one with stripes.
10. The sales lady was very helpful.
11. That hat is too expensive.
12. Where is the record department?
13. My feet are beginning to hurt.
14. Let's go to the coffee shop for a bite to eat.
15. Let's leave now and avoid the traffic rush.

SHORT STORIES

Mistaken Identity

When Julie offered to take care of a friend's dog for a few days, her husband was working the night shift. At the time, they were living in a trailer park. The dog, a large German shepherd called Bill, could not adjust his size and exuberance to the smaller trailer. Each time the door was opened he dashed outside. When Julie's mother visited, she found that the dog has been firmly tied to a post outside. "What's with Bill?" she said.

Julie gave her a weary look. "That dog," she said, "has ruined my reputation. Last night about ten o'clock he got loose and started running through the trailer park. I went after him shouting *Bill, Bill, come back!* Now, everybody here knows my husband's name is David," she sighed, "and that he works nights."

Questions

1. Where did Julie live?
2. What time did her husband work?
3. What did she offer to do?
4. What kind of dog was Bill?
5. How did he adjust to the trailer?
6. Who came to visit Julie?
7. Where was Bill?
8. At what time did Bill get loose?
9. What did Julie do?
10. What was the result?

Honesty — the Best Policy

"Ethics are vital to the successful businessman," said the man to a friend. The two men were just leaving to go to lunch.

"To give you an example, an old customer paid his account today with a hundred dollar bill. As he was leaving, I discovered that he had mistakenly handed me two hundreds stuck together. Immediately the question of ethics arose. Should I tell my partner or not?"

Shopping Problem

In the supermarket, last Saturday I noticed a young lady pushing a grocery cart filled to the top with groceries. When she was ready to check out, there were five check out lanes, but only one checker on duty. Unfortunately, there were about ten people in line ahead of her.

"I won't wait that long," she mumbled. "Let him take me out to dinner." So she pushed her shopping cart aside and walked out of the store empty-handed.

Have your helper make up questions once you have understood the story.

Change of Heart

Mr. Gilbert, who is hard-of-hearing, had to enter the hospital for some minor surgery. He was lucky in getting an excellent nurse for his room. One day when she was getting his bath for him, she said pleasantly, "I wish I had a million patients like you."

"I'm sorry. What did you say?" said Mr. Gilbert.

The nurse repeated for him, using a louder voice. "I wish I had a million patients like you."

"I still don't hear you. Would you please repeat it?" asked Mr. Gilbert.

The nurse, still louder now, but lacking her former enthusiasm, replied, "I wish I had a *dozen* patients like you."

Have your helper make up questions once you have understood the story.

Fair Trade

A man was walking down Madison Avenue one morning. During his stroll, he passed a pair of odd-looking fellows and overheard the pair discussing a cute little dog one of them was taking for its morning walk.

"Oh, what a cute little pup," commented one.

"I got it for my wife," beamed the other.

"How'd you ever make a trade like that?"

――――――

Cat and Mouse

A salesman stood sadly at the door of a farmhouse.

"I hate to tell you this, madam," he said, "but I just ran over your cat. I'm terribly sorry and I would like to replace him."

"Well, don't just stand there!" she snapped. "There's a mouse in the kitchen!"

――――――

Paying Guest

While stopping at a hotel, a man asked for some stationery to write a letter and the clerk inquired, "Are you a guest at the hotel?"

"No," answered the man indigantly. "I am *not* a guest. I am paying thirty dollars a day!"

1. List the environmental noise you have analyzed for pitch, loudness, and quality. Describe those noises using the three attributes just mentioned.

2. Make a note of the characteristics of your own voice and other people's voices (pitch, loudness, and quality).

Chapter V

AUDITORY TRAINING —
BACKGROUND NOISE

In Chapter IV, you were instructed to make note of the pitch, loudness, and quality of other people's voices. Now you should begin to monitor your own voice for those three characteristics. People with hard-of-hearing problems may either begin to speak too softly or begin shouting. To prevent yourself from doing either of these things, it is necessary for you to learn to listen to your own voice. A small tape recorder will be very helpful in this practice effort. By paying constant attention to the sound of your voice, you should be able to maintain not only a normal loudness level, but also a normal pitch. Besides the clues you get from listening, signs of tension of the throat and lower part of the face may also indicate that you are speaking too loudly and with too high a pitch. Make notes concerning the pitch, loudness, and quality of the voice you are using.

Continue to listen to the pitch, loudness, and quality of other people's voices, as explained in the last chapter. Have your helper speak and read to you using different levels of loudness and pitch and note which levels appear most satisfactory to you. By now your helper can vary the distance between the two of you for listening practice. Sometimes he can be close, at other times he could move to a farther part of the room or walk around the room reading or speaking to you. You should also begin listening practice in a small group of two or three people. Remember to fix your gaze on the face of the current speaker.

LISTENING WITH BACKGROUND NOISE

The speech-reader must learn to cope with background noise which may interfere with the understanding of speech. Therefore, part of the lesson should be given against a background of noise, so that he may learn to "fade it out." Some hard-of-hearing people find that they understand speech better in noisy places, and so do not need such practice. Types of background noise to be used may be:

1. TV
2. Radio
3. Records
4. Air conditioner
5. Refrigerator
6. Vacuum cleaner

The speech-reader is not asked about the content matter of the background noise. Rather he is to identify it and then learn to disregard it. The background noise should be just loud enough to distract the speech-reader. The helper should speak with as much voice as he would use in conversation with the normal hearing person when a similar amount of noise is present.

For these practice lessons a small tape recorder will be helpful. Speech items should be recorded against various levels and types of environmental noises. Understanding of the speech material can be tested by asking the speech-reader questions about the test material while the background noise is being played.

Further drills can be done to develop your ability to concentrate on the speech of the primary speaker. This skill will be very helpful to you in a noisy environment or when listening in a group of two or more individuals. This lesson can be done by having your helper read a list of test sentences, while at the same time a tape-recorded list of sentences is played in the background. During the time both the material that is tape-recorded and the material that is being read is presented to the speech-reader, he will be instructed to shift his attention to either the recorded material or the material being read by the helper. Soon the speech-reader's ability to concentrate on speech material will be enhanced. Because of the intense concentration required, which is usually quite tiring, this work should be done initially for only a few minutes at the close of each session. This type of work, being an advanced exercise, should be given only when the speech-reader is becoming more proficient in a quiet setting.

In the previous chapters, work has been given for you to identify environmental noises. This was done for two main reasons. One was to help you to learn to listen attentively and distinguish the differences between sounds as a preliminary to discrimination of more complex speech sounds. The other was to reduce the amount of distraction noise affords while listening to speech. Once sounds have been learned and discriminated, an individual is no longer as distracted by them and can tend to suppress them so that they *fade* into the background. This allows for better understanding of speech in a noisy situation. This is what the normal hearing person does, and what you can also do, especially as you become used to your hearing aid.

INCREASING TOLERANCE FOR SOUNDS

Some individuals who wear hearing aids have "recruitment" (the abnormally rapid growth of loudness); others are simply accustomed to sound being very faint. These people need training to increase their tolerance for sounds. If a person has a reduced dynamic range, in other words, a small distance between the threshold of detection and the threshold of discomfort, it is important that we attempt to broaden that range.

You should, over a period of training sessions, present training material first at a level of loudness that the speech-reader indicates as being comfortable, then the material should be presented at slightly higher levels. Soon you will find that the speech-reader will accept more and more increase in loudness during the training sessions. It is important that these changes in loudness be only small changes. Large upsetting changes will not increase understanding and perhaps only cause painful distractions. The result of such training will be to allow the individual to wear his hearing aid on a slightly higher volume setting and in doing so he will increase his understanding of speech.

HOW TO USE THE SENTENCES BASED
ON HOMOPHENOUS WORDS

"Homophenous" means "like-appearing." Homophenous words contain combinations of sounds that look exactly alike, as the organs of speech move in a similar manner to make them. For example "Pay," "Bay," and "May" look the same because the three sounds of P, B, and M contain similar movements. Homophenous words are distinguished from one another through speech reading only when they are spoken in context. The correct word is then understood from the meaning of the sentence:

"Shall I pay the bill?"
"The room has a bay window."
"This is the first of May."

The three words mentioned above are readily distinguished in the context of the sentences just given.

When practicing homophenous (look alike) words, the speech-reader should first be given a simple explanation, such as above. He should also know which homophenous words are to be used. But he should not know which word is to be used in a particular sentence. This aim is to train him to get the word from the meaning of the sentence.

Show the speech-reader the homophenous words. Choose any sentence in the group containing one of those words and say it. The speech-reader should then indicate which word was used. Repeat this procedure using other words in the group until all the sentences have been completed.

This chapter also contains exercises for sentences, conversational drills, and stories. Follow the procedure outlined in Chapter III for these exercises.

Group I Sentences

1. *my* My book is on the desk.
Where is my coat?
Do you have my keys?

2. *peach* We had peach pie for dessert.
The peach trees are in blossom.
Would you like an apricot or a peach?

3. *toy* That's an expensive toy.
Stop banging on that toy drum.
Let's go to the toy department.

4. *bay* We went fishing on the bay.
The bay is good for swimming.
Is your yacht club on the bay?

5. *home* What time will you be home?
My home is in California.
How far is it to your home?

6. *ham* Let's have ham and eggs for breakfast.
We had cold ham and turkey for supper.
I think I'll have a ham sandwich.

7. *farm* The farm is thirty miles from the city.
Do you like living on the farm?
The farm house is very old.

Group II Sentences

1. The office party will last till eight o'clock.
   Why is the office so dark today?
   The office should run smoother today.

2. I would like to examine the interesting rocks.
   To examine you completely, I must look in your mouth.
   Examine the evidence closely, to be sure you are correct.

3. I will close the window to the kitchen.
   The smell is coming from the kitchen.
   The kitchen is always the warmest room in the house.

4. Hold on to your kite, or it'll blow away.
   Why don't you paint a face on your kite?
   The kite got tangled in the trees.

5. Do you have a comb?
   My comb is on the dressing table.
   Did you comb your hair?

6. So you have some money?
   Some of my books are missing.
   "You can fool some of the people, some of the time."

7. I dropped my pencil.
   My pencil broke in the middle of my test.
   Just pencil in the correct answer and you will get credit.

8. Yesterday I bought a new and expensive typewriter.
   This typewriter is a self-correcting model.
   We got a new typewriter for our secretary.

9. I used a 35mm camera to take these pictures.
   This camera is relatively simple to learn how to use.
   The camera shop was out of the type of film I needed.

10. The doctor may need to operate if it doesn't heal.
    It is a very difficult piece of equipment to operate.
    To operate the machines you have to turn this switch on
    first.

11. The pajamas were making me itch.
    I must have very soft material for my pajamas.

I almost forgot to pack my pajamas.

12. His education limited him from getting a good job.
A quality education is an important asset in our modern society.
He did not have much formal education but was a truly knowledgeable person.

13. The umbrella will surely stop the rain.
The wind prevented me from opening my umbrella.
If my umbrella is broken, may I use yours?

14. My mustache makes me look years older.
It is difficult to keep the mustache clean.
If I don't trim my mustache it becomes too difficult to take care of.

Group III Sentences

1. Yesterday I bought a new and expensive typewriter.
   It should make it easier for us to type our reports.

2. I used a 35mm camera to take these pictures.
   They all seem very clear and have excellent color.

3. The doctor may need to operate if it doesn't heal.
   But he hopes that everything will heal properly.

4. The pajamas were making me itch.
   I will have to take them back to the store.

5. The umbrella will surely stop the rain.
   I plan to wear my good suit even if it rains.

6. His lack of education limited him from getting a good job.
   Unfortunately he has the most experience and would be the best at the job.

7. My mustache makes me look years older.
   I don't have any plans to cut it off.

HOMOPHENOUS WORDS
(look-alike words)

Pay — Bay — May

1. What do they pay you?
2. Friday is pay day.
3. You usually have to pay for what you want.

1. The bay is very good for fishing.
2. We went sailing on the bay.
3. The house has bay windows.

1. May is usually a pleasant month.
2. May I borrow your pen.
3. "April showers bring May flowers."

Park — Bark — Mark

1. The street was too crowded to park the car.
2. Let's go for a walk in the park.
3. The park is pleasant in the Spring.

1. His bark is worse than his bite.
2. The tree was beginning to shed its bark.
3. The dog's bark scared the little boy.

1. I'll put a mark on the page for you.
2. Did you get a good mark in English?
3. Mark my words.

PHRASE CONVERSATIONAL DRILL

About Sports

1. Fly ball
2. Free throw
3. Touchdown
4. Forward pass
5. Great catch
6. Field goal
7. Popcorn and peanuts
8. Strike three
9. Bases loaded
10. A triple play
11. Bad call by the umpire
12. Fast runner on first
13. Head for the showers
14. Half time show
15. Seventh inning stretch

SENTENCE CONVERSATIONAL DRILL

At Home

1. There's someone at the door.
2. The phone's ringing.
3. Were there any letters today?
4. Please turn down the TV, it's too loud.
5. What's for supper?
6. I think we need new rugs.
7. The washing machine is broken.
8. Please clean up your room, it's a mess.
9. We're having company for supper.
10. The man has come to cut the lawn.
11. Where will I plant these bushes?
12. Don't let your ashes fall on the carpet.
13. Switch on the lights.
14. Let's change the furniture in the family room.
15. Please turn off the air conditioner.

Practice Lip Reading the Following

1. Names of food and drinks
2. Names of flowers and shrubs
3. Furniture in your home
4. Names of TV programs and TV stars
5. Names of appliances, tools, and utensils
6. Names of books, magazines, and newspapers

SENTENCE CONVERSATIONAL DRILL

Numbers and Figures

1. The number of our house is 418.
2. The train is six minutes late.
3. Our phone number is 317-9264.
4. I'll be about a half hour late.
5. You're running ten minutes early.
6. It takes forty-five minutes to drive to the city.
7. Our family room is twenty feet by fifteen feet.
8. The apartment has six rooms and two baths.
9. He has just turned twenty-one.
10. We all need a holiday on January 1st.
11. I'll be back in ten minutes.
12. The book department is on the fifth floor.
13. My father is six feet, two inches tall.
14. My sister weighs 120 pounds.
15. Did you say the date was the 27th?

SHORT STORIES

Golfer's Heaven

An avid golfer who finally got to heaven found one championship course after another. One approach was covered with tall fir trees and really looked tough. Someone was attempting to drive a ball 400 yards over the thickest clump of trees.

"Who does he think he is?" asked the newcomer. "St. Peter?"

"He *is* St. Peter," whispered an angel in the gallery. "Trouble is, he thinks he's Jack Nicklaus."

Old Baldy

Johnny was looking through the family photograph album.

"Say, Mom," he asked, "who's this curly-headed guy in this picture?"

His mother looked. "That's your father, Johnny," she said.

Johnny looked puzzled for a few minutes. Then he asked, "Then who's that bald-headed guy upstairs?"

Golfer's Day Off

At breakfast, Mr. Smith suddenly announced that he didn't have to go to the office that morning.

"Listen," said his wife, "don't think you're going to run off and play golf today and leave me with all this work."

"Golf is the furthest thing from my mind," the husband protested. "And will you please pass the putter?"

Big Baseball Score

A man stopped to watch a Little League baseball game and

asked a youngster named Robby, what the score was.

"We're behind, 18 to 0," was the answer.

"Well," said the man, "I must say you don't look discouraged."

"Discouraged?" Robby said puzzled. "Why should we be discouraged? We haven't come to bat yet."

Baseball Sickness

A note was left by a ten-year-old boy named Rusty, for his mother, who was shopping when he got home from school. "I have a very bad headache and a stomachache. I have taken two aspirins and a glass of milk and gone out to play baseball."

The Big Trade

A little boy came home from playing ball with a disgusted look on his face. When his father asked him what was wrong, he replied, "I was traded."

"That shouldn't make you feel bad," said the father. "All baseball players get traded."

"I know," answered the boy. "But I was traded for a glove."

PTA Meeting

At a PTA meeting the dean of the school started to say, "It's as simple as two and two are four." He hesitated and then turned to the English teacher sitting at his side and said, "Pardon me, Mr. Jones, I suppose I should say two and two *is* four?"

"Don't ask me," came the retort. "I'm not a math teacher."

The Big Sale

A department store was having a sale on yard goods. The crowd of women pushed around the table where there was a ten-yard limit on some fine materials. Soon a woman complained to the manager that she had been shoved out of line by another woman. Pointing a finger at the offender, the manager said to a sales girl, "Penalize that woman five yards!"

I Didn't Hear You, Officer

The motorcycle policeman waved the motorist over to the side of the road. When they had both stopped, the officer walked to the car and said very angrily, "How come you didn't stop back there when I blew my whistle, and later when I went after you and sounded my siren?"

"I'm sorry, officer," said the motorist, "but I didn't hear you. I must be getting hard-of-hearing."

"Well, don't worry about that," said the officer sarcastically. "You'll be getting your hearing in court, tomorrow morning!"

Truth Will Out

Paul Wilson, a private in the Army, had just been transferred to a new base. The billeting sergeant there had a system of putting all troublemakers on the first floor. There he could watch them himself.

As Pvt. Wilson stood at attention, the sergeant asked, "Do you go to church on Sunday?"

"Yes."

"Do you write your parents regularly?"

"Yes."

"Do you drink, or stay up late, play cards, and listen to music all night?"

"No."

The sergeant nodded pleasantly and seemed pleased with the answers. Then turning to his clerk he said, "He's a liar. Put him on the first floor."

———

Have your helper make up questions about the story.

SHORT STORIES

Ask Questions First

A department of motor vehicles examiner stepped into a car which was stopped at the curb. All of the cars were in line to take their driving tests. He went through the usual safety checks with the brakes, lights, and turn indicators. The driver followed each instruction without a word. They pulled into traffic.

"Turn right," ordered the examiner.

"Turn left . . . . . now stop . . . . . go back . . . . . now make a right turn and then back up."

Each order was followed perfectly. Finally after about fifteen minutes, the driver asked, "Do you mind telling me what this is all about? I'm from out of town and I just pulled to the curb to check my road map."

————

Renovations

After a period of several months of urging from my teenage daughter Mary, I finally decided to dress more fashionably and "up to date." I went downtown to a boutique and bought a boldly patterned miniskirt. I also bought yellow stockings to complete the outfit.

A few days later my husband and I were invited to a barbecue. However, I didn't show him my new outfit; I hid it under a coat. I thought I would surprise him and my friends at the barbecue with the new me.

When we arrived, I flung my coat off and a startled look crossed my husband's face. Then taking me by the hand, he addressed the guests, "Well you see, I couldn't afford a new wife, so I had the old one slip covered."

————

1. Make a note of your successes while listening and speech reading your helper, when a background noise is present.

2. Make notes concerning your reaction to listening and speech reading in small groups of people. What were the difficulties you encountered, and what success did you have?

Chapter VI

ADVANCED AUDITORY TRAINING
AND SPEECH READING

By now, you should be combining speech reading with auditory training to gain the maximum benefit during communication. Any previous exercises which proved difficult should be repeated before doing the work outlined in this chapter.

SPEECH READING FOR DIFFICULT SITUATIONS

For many people with a hearing loss, understanding speech in groups is always a difficult situation. To help improve this, have your helper review the exercise in the previous chapters by speaking to you from varying distances and different angles. Train yourself to watch the speaker at all times. At first do this in a quiet setting. When you feel proficient at this, begin practicing with a small group of two to three people and gradually increase the number over successive weeks. Keep your gaze focused on the current speaker's face, and try to find out the general meaning of what is being said. It is a good idea when joining a group to find out the general topic of conversation, as this will help you understand what is being said.

In order to help you understand speech while listening to a speaker against a background noise, review the drill material using the noises previously suggested. At first practice with just one person who should face you when speaking. When you become proficient at this, have the speaker partially hide his face or move around while talking. Finally, practice listening against a noise background with small groups of two or three people.

This chapter contains further assignments for you, plus additional ideas for practicing "look alike" words and conversational drills. Also included are a number of sentences for advanced speech reading and auditory training, containing a choice of two words both of which fit the meaning of the sentence. The helper should show the two words which are in brackets, and then, choosing one, read the sentence to the listener. The speech-reader has to decide which word was read. These sentences differ from the ones used for homophenous words in that either word is applicable in the context; therefore the sentences are more difficult than the previous exercises. Also, there are three auditory training sounds tables which describe the visibility of speech sounds. These tables may be used for speech reading and auditory training practice as described on Table I. Continue speech reading practice by the discussion of articles, TV programs or movies you have seen. Aim for daily practice periods and try to apply what you have learned in everyday situations.

LIP READING — AUDITORY TRAINING SOUND CHART
MOST VISIBLE SOUNDS
TABLE I

consonants	b	p	m	w	j	ch	sh
	beet	peal	meal	we'll	jean	cheat	she'll
	bill	pill	mill	will	Jill	chill	shill
	bale	pail	mail	wail	jail	chain	shale
	bell	pell	mell	well	jell	Chet	shell
	bat	pal	mat	wal	Jan	chat	shall
		pot	moll	wad	jot		shot
	ball	Paul	maul	wall	jaunt		shawl
	bowl	pole	mole		Joel		shoal
	bull	pull		wool			should
	boot	pool	moot	wound	jewel		shoot
	bulb	pulp	mull	what	jut		shut
	burn	pearl	Merle	whirl		churl	shirt

Have your helper read the words down the columns so that you may learn to distinguish by listening and speech reading the different vowel sounds. Then have your helper read across the columns for you to distinguish the difference between the consonant sounds. Repeat this procedure using the charts of the medium and least visible sounds. Also, let your helper place the words in sentences, and see if you can distinguish which word is used.

LIP READING — AUDITORY TRAINING SOUND CHART
MEDIUM VISIBILITY SOUNDS
TABLE II

consonants	v	f	th	d	t	n	l	z	s
	veal	feal		deal	teal	kneel	lead	zeal	seal
		fill	thin	dill	till	nil	Lil		sill
	vale	fail	they'll	dale	tail	nail	late	Zale	sail
	Vet	fell	then	dell	tell	knell	let	Zen	sell
	vat	fat	that	Dad	tan	gnat	lad		sat
				doll	tot	knot	lot	zot	Sol
	vault	fall		dawn	tall	naught	loll		Saul
	vote	foal		dole	toll	knoll	loan	zone	soul
		full							soot
		fool	Thule	duel	tool	Nuel	loot	zoot	Seoul
		fun	thud	dull	ton	nut	lull		sun
		furl	third	dirt	turn	knurl	learn		

LIP READING — AUDITORY TRAINING SOUND CHART
LEAST VISIBLE SOUNDS
TABLE III

consonants	g	k	h	y	r
		keel	heel	ye'll	real
	gill	kill	hill		rill
	gale	kale	hale	Yale	rail
	get	Ken	hell	yell	red
	gat	Cal	Hal		rat
	got	cot	hot	yacht	rot
	gall	call	hall	y'all	Raul
	goal	coal	hole		roll
	good	could	hood		
	ghoul	cool	hoot	Yule	rule
	gull	cull	hull		rut
	girl	curl	hurl	yearn	

Group I Sentences

1. *star*   The stars are all out tonight.
Did you see the movie star?
"Star light, star bright, first star I've seen tonight."

2. *shore*   We found these shells down by the shore.
The shore front was damaged by the storm.
The boys were building a sand castle down by the shore.

3. *dish*   Put the plates in the dishwasher.
Don't break that dish.
This dish is a family heirloom.

4. *wife*   I've invited the boss and his wife for supper.
My wife can't manage her checking account.
He bought his wife a new car.

5. *coat*   Is that a new coat?
I like that sport coat over there.
Put on a coat, it's cold outside.

6. *paper*   Will you bring in the paper?
I think we'll use paper dishes for the party.
Did you see the advertisement for the dress made out of paper?

7. *coffee* I like my coffee strong and black.
Put the coffee in the coffee pot.
Did you remember to buy some coffee?

Group II Sentences

1. I had my purse stolen in the store.
   How do you get so much in your purse?
   That purse matches my gloves.

2. They're building a new church.
   Did you go to church last Sunday?
   That was an interesting church service.

3. That book is on the best seller list.
   I don't understand why they banned that book.
   Who has taken my book?

4. The waitress gave me some crackers with my lunch.
   Nothing tastes quite as good as peanut butter on crackers.
   People on diets often eat soup and crackers.

5. The Scotch™ tape held the paper together.
   I put Scotch tape on the book to cover up the torn page.
   If we run out of Scotch tape, be sure to order some more.

6. The chart was complete before the client came today.
   I already put your name in the chart.
   The chart recorded how often you should take the medicine.

7. I was reporting on your case just as the doctor came in.
   Reporting the news everyday is a difficult and time-consuming job.
   I am reporting to you because you are in charge of this job.

8. There was a lot of movement in the audience.
   I didn't see any movement in the woods.
   Stop the movement while I study.

9. The downstairs apartment has three bedrooms.
   Go downstairs and clear up the living room.
   I went downstairs late last night for something to eat.

10. Do you remember when we went shopping last week?
    I don't remember that trip.
    I remember the time we all had a party at the lake.

11. The furniture is too heavy for me to move.

I hope the colors will match our furniture.

Don't forget to move the furniture when you vacuum.

12. It will be a challenge to finish in the top half of my class.

If you challenge him he will play the game.

The challenge match will attract a large crowd.

13. I use the dictionary when I write my papers.

If people would use the dictionary, they would learn a lot more.

It is sometimes difficult to find all the words in the dictionary.

14. Our neighbor will watch our house while we are gone.

My neighbor doesn't cut his lawn.

My neighbor came to borrow a cup of sugar.

Group III Sentences

1. There was a lot of movement in the audience.
   The chairman had to ask the audience to take their seats.

2. The downstairs apartment has three bedrooms.
   With your family you will need the extra room.

3. Do you remember when we went shopping last week?
   I thought we would never find the dress you wanted.

4. The furniture is too heavy for me to move.
   We'll have to wait for the moving van.

5. It will be a challenge to finish in the top half of my class.
   If I can do it, it should help me get into college.

6. I use the dictionary when I write my papers.
   The dictionary improves my papers and increases my vocabulary.

7. Our neighbor will watch our house while we are gone.
   We will only be gone for two weeks.

HOMOPHENOUS WORDS
(look-alike words)

Tea — Tee — Knee

1. Would you like a cup of tea?
2. Do you take your tea with or without sugar?
3. I like lemon in my tea.

1. Are you ready to tee off yet?
2. I'll meet you on the first tee.
3. Why are they taking so long to tee off?

1. He cut his knee when he fell over.
2. She was knee deep in work.
3. I can't bend my right knee.

Flower — Flour

1. We have both a flower and a vegetable garden.
2. What kind of flower is that?
3. Put the flowers in the vase.

1. Sift the flour before you measure it.
2. I want five pounds of flour.
3. She spilled the flour all over the kitchen floor.

Further Homophenous Words to Practice

1. beach	beech	peach
2. belt	pelt	melt
3. path	bath	math
4. wash	watch	
5. weak	week	
6. wait	wade	weight
7. win	wind	wit
8. which	wish	
9. card	cart	guard
10. ear	here	hear
11. save	safe	
12. ship	chip	
13. mash	match	batch
14. wood	would	
15. hall	all	haul

Have your helper make up sentences similar to those previously described for practice of these homophenous words.

PHRASE CONVERSATIONAL DRILL

About Eating

1. I'm hungry
2. Set the table
3. Dry the glasses
4. Drink your milk
5. Carve the turkey
6. Pass the salt
7. More meat, please
8. No more, thanks
9. I'm getting full
10. Great food
11. No dessert for me
12. Excuse me
13. Finish your potatoes
14. Help with the dishes
15. I'll wash — you dry

SENTENCE CONVERSATIONAL DRILL

About Relatives

1. My mother is a wonderful cook.
2. Have you any brothers and sisters?
3. Where is your father working now?
4. My mother-in-law is visiting us again.
5. Has your son graduated yet?
6. Our daughter has just entered college.
7. Grandfather is a veteran of World War I.
8. I wish grandma wouldn't spoil the children so much.
9. Stop arguing with your sister.
10. My son-in-law has turned hippie.
11. I'm going north to visit my uncle and aunt.
12. My older brother is in the Army.
13. My niece is living with us.
14. How old is your sister?

SENTENCE CONVERSATIONAL DRILL

On the Airplane

1. We waited in line about ten minutes.
2. The man at the ticket counter told us we would have a thirty-minute wait before boarding the plane.
3. At the coffee shop we ordered a light snack.
4. While boarding the plane the stewardess told us what seats we were to sit in.
5. Our seats were toward the front of the plane.
6. After we were seated, the no smoking sign came on.
7. We had to keep our seatbelts on for a few minutes.
8. During the flight the stewardess gave us refreshments.
9. The view from the plane was breathtaking.
10. The cartoons they showed were very amusing.
11. The landing at the airport was very smooth.
12. The stewardess was polite throughout the entire trip.
13. It was a nice surprise to have our relatives greet us at the gate.
14. I hope we won't have trouble getting our luggage.
15. I had a very pleasant flight, but it is nice to be home.

SENTENCE CONVERSATIONAL DRILL

At the Movies

1. There's a double feature at the theater tonight.
2. It will take us about twenty minutes to get there.
3. If we leave now, we should be there for the beginning of the feature.
4. You go buy the tickets, while I park the car.
5. Would you like some popcorn or a soft drink?
6. Let's sit in the middle, about halfway down.
7. Stop talking, the movie is about to start.
8. I'll go get us a drink before the intermission is over.
9. So far the movie has been very exciting.
10. I always enjoy these detective movies.
11. He's one of my favorite actors.
12. Their costumes are very authentic.
13. I'm getting sleepy, I hope I can stay awake through the next film.
14. I always enjoy seeing the coming attractions.
15. Let's plan to go again next week.

Further Topics for Practice in
Conversational Drill

Back seat driving
At the garage
About holidays
At the drug store
About magazines
At the restaurant
At the back
At election time
At the post office
At a party
Proverbs and sayings
Space travel

Advanced Speech Reading and
Auditory Training Sentences

To the Helper — Read the sentences using only one or the other of the word pair choices.

To the listener — You will need to use both your lip reading and auditory training in order to get the correct word said, as each word fits the meaning.

1. She began to (heat — eat) the beans.
2. Who will (close — clothe) them when we are gone?
3. The girl removed the (can — pan) from the fire.
✓4. She looked at the (nice — knife) fork and spoon.
5. He was asked to look the (will — well) over.
6. She put the chicken in the (pen — pan) and replaced the cover.
7. Her skin color was (not — nut) brown.
8. He (taught — caught) the children without effort.
9. He explained the role to the (fool — full).
✓10. The child liked to (swing — swim) for hours.
11. I have (run — won) this race many times.
✓12. (Wet — let) your hair down, and come with me.
13. He traveled along the winding dusty (rail — trail).
14. He broke the (rock — lock) with a sledgehammer.
15. The (rows — rays) of lights were still visible to the west.
✓16. He gazed at the bright (shine — sign).
17. The (cut — cat) was quite a nuisance.
18. The wine tasted (bitter — better) today.
✓19. The Rangers examined the condition of the (park — bark).
20. The mountaineer stopped and felt his (back — pack).

Advanced Speech Reading and
Auditory Training Sentences

 1. Will you (lead — read) the way, please.
 2. The (patter — packer) could be heard down the hallway.
 3. I think they will put a (bun — ban) on those plates.
 4. The sun will (heat — hit) the patio early today.
 5. He gripped the (tap — top) and turned it.
 6. The shiny new (bead — bed) was just what the girl wanted.
 7. The (cot — cat) always seemed to be in the way.
 8. She talked without a (pause — cause) on into the night.
 9. A (life — wife) without humor can mean gloom for a man.
10. When you complete that last page, it will be (done — dawn).
11. How many do you think you can (fell — sell) in a day?
12. The (row — low) boat just barely made it.
13. Soak it in the (brine — brown) vat for an hour.
14. I think you can (close — clothe) the baby in this room.
15. He heard a loud (bus — buzz) below him.
16. It is important to choose the right (ray — way) at this point.
17. All we lack is (tin — ten) for our production.
18. I'm quitting, the (sum — sun) is too much for me.
19. The card in your hand is (nine — mine).
20. Why don't you try to (sit — fit) in sideways?

Advanced Speech Reading and
Auditory Training Sentences

1. The (wind — wink) was a big factor in the outcome.
2. The (girls — curls) proved to be very difficult to straighten out.
3. The success of the operation depended on the next (development — envelopment).
4. Be sure you put in the (right — light) package.
5. How did you ever get that (match — much).
6. The sudden (wedding — wetting) was a shock.
7. The crime was averted by the (scream — screen).
8. He shuddered at the thought of the approaching (night — might).
9. It says in the instructions we can use (ether — either).
10. The (sore — shore) needed to be cleaned up.
11. The critic thought the word (clothe — clove) had been overused.
12. He decided to (break — rake) no more than ten minutes.
13. Put it in with the (latter — ladder).
14. I was told that I had better not (sing — sin) again.
15. The climber was determined to (dare — bear) the dangers of the mountain.
16. The (boat — bout) was well worth waiting for.
17. The student realized he could not longer (breeze — breathe) in as easily as before.
18. The new (wing — ring) was a gorgeous sight to behold.
19. He looked in every one of his coats for the lost (pin — pen).
20. If you apply yourself you can show (fast — vast) improvement.

Advanced Speech Reading and
Auditory Training Sentences

1. The new (grain — crane) was the best he'd seen in years.
2. He had had all the (zeal — veal) he could take for now.
3. He explained that the information was (tentative — sensitive).
4. She found herself surrounded by (bays — boys).
5. Please try to buy a (sheath — sheaf) for me.
6. Put the shirt in the (seam — same) repair bin.
7. He looked forward to getting his (wings — rings).
8. The old man checked the (trap — track) carefully.
9. The (hair — air) was hot and dry.
10. There is too much (lead — red) in that brand.
11. This is the way to get a good (tune — tone).
12. The (fire — fair) started on Saturday.
13. If you (heat — hit) the wall first, you'll have a better result.
14. He opened the pen door and quickly (shot — shut) it.
15. What is the (rate — late) charge on that order?
16. He hoped to be able to go to the right (place — plays).
17. He remembered the evil (look — luck) the medicine man had given him.
18. It all hinges on how many you (cook — took).
19. The man traveled far trying to find a lost (soul — seal).
20. (Pool — pull) your resources together would be my advice.

**Advanced Speech Reading and
Auditory Training Sentences
(Involving High Frequency Sounds)**

1. These sentences involve words differing only in their high frequency sounds which are often confused.

   a. *Toll*   All of the travelers have to use the new toll road.

      Dole   The mothers will dole out one piece of candy a day to each child.

      Pole   The telephone pole was put up just ten feet from our house.

      Bowl   The athletes all want to play in the Super Bowl.

   b. *Bin*   The bin was completely filled with grain.

      Pin   Mother stuck the straight pin in her finger.

      Tin   The tin plate was put over the electrical wires.

   c. *Kill*   The frightened lady asked the man to kill the snake.

      Gill   The teacher pointed out the fish's gill to the class.

      Cot   The army cot was not very comfortable.

      Got   I got home in plenty of time for dinner.

      Cane   My grandfather uses a cane when he goes for a walk.

      Gain   What do you hope to gain from that?

   d. *Kin*   All my kin will be at the party.

      Fin   The fin could be seen from the shore.

      Sin   He asked forgiveness for his sin.

      Shin   The man hit his shin on the table leg.

      Chin   The little boy had a dimple on his chin.

      Thin   The thin man was called for the police lineup.

   e. *Fat*   Don't include much fat in your diet.

      Vat   The hot grease was put in the large vat.

      That   That store will be closed on Sunday.

   f. *Those*   Those boys will have to stay after school.

      Foes   Our families have been foes over this problem for years.

   g. *File*   I will ask the secretary to file those charts.

    Vile   The school board member said the book contained vile language.

h. *Sue*   We may need to sue the company.

   Zoo   The zoo animals were all hungry.

i. *Some* Some children need more discipline.

   Thumb While slicing the tomato, I cut my thumb.

2. These sentences involve words differing in medium frequency sounds, often confused.

   a. *Hum*   He started to hum the song he heard on the radio.

      Hun   The Hun tribe was a warlike group of people.

      Hung   The picture hung in the hallway.

   b. *Run*   I will run the campaign myself.

     Rum   The drink was full of rum.

     Rung   The doorbell was rung a number of times.

   c. *Ram*   The ram was an active, aggressive animal.

     Ran   I ran around the track twice.

     Rang   The doorbell rang three times before the host came.

   d. *Yet*   I can't go to school yet.

     Let   Let us go home before it gets too dark.

     Wet   The wet streets are dangerous.

   e. *Young* Young men need to look for good jobs.

     Lung   His lung capacity was not great.

     Rung   The telephone was rung too many times.

   f. *Yap*   The little dog will yap if we leave him alone.

     Lap   Come sit in my lap so I can rock you to sleep.

     Rap   We all sat around the fire to rap about our day.

   g. *Yacht* The yacht was large and expensive.

     Lot   Don't sell the lot yet, I hope to buy it.

     Rot   Don't let the vegetables rot in the garden.

     Watt   We need a 75 watt light bulb for that lamp.

3. Vowel discrimination

   a. *Read*   Can you read the book tonight?

     Rid   Get rid of the company, it's getting late.

     Raid   The raid was over before darkness came.

b. *Pet*   My pet was thirsty and hungry when I came home.

Pat   Pat the dog on his head.

Pot   Pot the plants in good, rich soil.

c. *Saw*   I saw you get on the plane.

So   I came back to finish the work so I can get paid.

Sue   If we need to sue, it will cost a lot of money.

Advanced Speech Reading and
Auditory Training Sentences
(Involving High Frequency Sounds)

1. After the fire the (peat — sheet) was still smoldering.
2. It will take another five minutes for it to be thoroughly (steeped — seeped).
3. The boys watched the baseball game through the (peep — peek) hole.
4. Because of the large field, a number of (sheets — heats) were required.
5. A blow to the (cheek — sheik) was what started all the trouble.
6. Before you leave for the night, (heat — heap) up the coals.
7. After the vase crashed, the siamese kittens (peeked — peeped) out from behind the drapes.
8. Ride the (cheap — steep) one if you want to have some real fun.
9. The (cheat — sheep) moved reluctantly ahead of his captor's prodding.
10. The liquid will probably (keep — seep) for several days.
11. The (peach — speech) at lunch was unusually delightful.
12. She (seeks — seats) her pupils alphabetically.
13. Little (cheeps — peeps) could be heard coming from the nest.
14. Becoming red and flushed, the (cheeks — cheats) readily disclosed embarrassment.
15. The holiday (feats — feast) were remembered with much nostalgia.
16. When she (speaks — squeaks) everyone stops and listens.
17. Your mission is to (speak — seek) out, persuade and sign recruits.
18. While the owner is away, the neighbor (heaps — keeps) food in the dog's bowl.
19. Can you tell me what the record was in (skeet — feet)?
20. I'm glad to be back; it is really a wonderful (treat — street).

Advanced Speech Reading and
Auditory Training Sentences
(Involving High Frequency Sounds)

1. There is much more work needed to be done on the (kits — skits).
2. He said he did it for the (kiss — kicks).
3. I just like to (sit — sip) on it to relax me.
4. (Sis — Six) has the next turn coming up.
5. He hollered across the room, "How many (tipped — tips) today?"
6. The (tip — tick) was stuck and would not come out.
7. The (kit — kick) was delivered swiftly and came as quite a surprise.
8. She always (sips — skips) very daintily.
9. Everywhere he looked he saw (ticks — picks).
10. After a near miss, he responded with a (hit — hiss).
11. It appeared that the (pick — pit) had claimed another victim.
12. Gather up the (chicks — sticks) and let's be on our way.
13. Three years on the stage and she had never been (kissed — hissed).
14. As far as he was concerned, it was (fist — fixed) before the debate.
15. The dog just (sits — fits) in the dog house.
16. The man (sipped — skipped) it on the rocks.
17. His (hip — skip) seemed to be frequently out of place.
18. What was the most he had ever (kicked — picked)?
19. The judge was asked to make the penalty (stiff — stick).
20. (Fit — Fix) the valve in the old water line.

Practice Drill

This exercise is designed to help improve both your auditory training and speech reading ability. Your helper should choose one pair of sounds, show them to you, and then say them while you watch and listen. He should then show and say each pair of words, e.g. — few-chew, for you to repeat them back. Then he should choose one word of a pair and place it in a sentence. You watch and listen for the word and repeat the sentence back to him. When all pairs of words have been practiced, your helper should just say the words for you to repeat.

1. f & ch	2. sh & f	3. f & k	4. s & sh
few-chew	show-foe	fit-kit	lease-leash
fin-chin	shore-fore	four-core	sew-show
filed-child	shade-fade	find-kind	sigh-shy
calf-catch	cash-calf	cliff-click	sip-ship
four-chore	leash-leaf	laugh-lack	save-shave

5. p & f	6. ch & sh	7. t & p	8. f & s
pour-four	chop-shop	tail-pail	fine-sign
pile-file	chair-share	cat-cap	flat-slat
par-far	watch-wash	cut-cup	cuff-cuss
cap-calf	catch-cash	tar-par	knife-nice
cup-cuff	cheap-sheep	toll-pole	lift-list

9. th & f	10. t & th	11. k & t	12. k & p
thin-fin	tie-thigh	kick-tick	pike-pipe
thirst-first	tin-thin	kite-tight	car-par
three-free	trill-thrill	code-toad	crock-crop
thought-fought	mit-myth	shirk-shirt	cry-pry
thrill-frill	pat-path	park-part	coal-pole

13. f & t	14. s & z	15. th & s	16. p & b
four-tore	ice-eyes	theme-seam	pin-bin
fall-tall	seal-zeal	thin-sin	pie-buy

fan-tan	sip-zip	thumb-sum	pole-bowl
fill-till	loose-lose	truth-truce	cap-cab
free-tree	bus-buzz	thank-sank	rope-robe

SHORT STORIES

Flat Broke

A man called his creditors together to tell them that he was about to go into bankruptcy. "I owe you over $100,000," he said. "And my assets aren't enough to pay five cents on the dollar. So it will be impossible for you to get anything, unless you want to cut me up and divide me among you."

One creditor spoke up immediately. "I move we do it," he said. "I'd like to have his gall."

Shoe Repair

While rummaging through his attic, a man found a shoe repair ticket that was nine years old. Figuring that he had nothing to lose, he went to the shop and presented the ticket to the proprietor, who reluctantly began a search for the unclaimed shoes. After ten minutes, the owner reappeared and handed back the ticket.

"Well," asked the customer, "did you find the pair?"

"Yes," replied the shop owner. "They'll be ready Tuesday."

ESP

Last year, a course in extrasensory perception was taught at an eastern university. A sign on the classroom door read:

"ESP LAB — No need to knock — we know you're there!"

Football Widow

One of our neighbors is an avid football fan and spends every

Sunday afternoon in the fall before the TV set to watch the games. One Sunday just before the kickoff, his wife, who doesn't share his enthusiasm, was vacuuming the living room. Concerned that she would interfere with his reception, he asked what she was doing. She replied grimly, "I'm cleaning up the stadium!"

———

The Jolly Green Giant

The favorite costume of a Cleveland mother-to-be was a green maternity blouse over green slacks. She hadn't realized how often she's worn it until her TV-minded seven-year-old, seeing her approaching, called out, "Here comes the Jolly Green Giant!"

———

Repairmen's Problem

A gang of country road repairmen were way out in the country to fix a road when they discovered they had left their shovels back in town. They phoned the county engineer to report their problem.

"I'll send the shovels out right away," said the engineer. "Meanwhile, lean on each other."

———

Hospital Waiting Room

Three men were in the hospital waiting room when the nurse rushed in and said to the first man, "Sir, you're the father of twins."

"Hey, Isn't that a coincidence?" he replied. "I'm a member of the Minnesota Twins baseball team."

Later the nurse came in and said to the second man, "Sir, you're the father of triplets."

"Gee," the man exclaimed. "Another coincidence! I'm with the 3M Company."

The third man jumped to his feet, grabbed his hat and said, "I'm getting out of here. I work for 7 UP!"

Texas Boasting

"There is the Alamo," said the proud Texan to his friend from Boston.

"That ruin is where only 136 Texans held off 15,000 of Santa Ana's army for days. Did you ever have any heroes like that in Massachusetts?"

"Well, I should say we did!" answered the Bostonian. "We had Paul Revere, for example."

"Paul Revere!" snorted the Texan. "Do you mean that fellow who had to ride for help?"

The Raise

In asking for a raise, the employee hinted that several companies were after him.

"What companies?" his boss asked.

The man replied, "The gas company, electric company, finance company . . . . ."

Wife's Lament

A dutiful wife said plaintively, "I've sweltered at baseball games, I've shivered through football, I've been sunburned and mosquito-bitten on fishing trips. Why can't you be like other husbands and not take me anywhere?"

Father Knows Best

A son came to his father for some helpful discussion.

"Dad, what's an ocelot?"

"It's Sir Ocelot, son, and he was one of King Arthur's Knights of the Round Table."

"Dad, what's algebra?"

"It's the language the people speak in Algeria, son."

"Dad, what do they call people who live in Paris, France?"

"Parasites, son."

"Who was the father of our country?"

"I don't know son."

"Dad, you don't mind me asking you all these questions, do you?"

"Of course not, son, How else can you ever become educated?"

In Plain English Please

If you don't think plain English can be confusing how about this conversation, overheard in a hardware store.

"Do you have any four-volt, two-watt bulbs?"

"For what?"

"No, two."

"Two what?"

"Yes."

"No."

Life After Death

"Do you believe in life after death?" the boss asked one of his younger employees.

"Yes, sir."

"Well, then, that makes everything just fine," the boss went on. "About an hour after you left yesterday to go to your grandfather's funeral, he stopped by to see you."

Congressman's Wife

The Congressman's wife shook him vigorously in the middle of the night. "Wake up, John!" she whispered frantically. "There's a thief in the house!"

"No way," he replied. "In the Senate maybe. In the House — *never*."

Out of the Mouths of Babes

The little girl had just returned from Sunday School and was having dinner with her family. She asked her father when her baby brother would be able to talk.

"Oh, he won't talk until he's about two years old," said the father.

"That's too bad," said the little girl. "It was much better in the olden days when babies could talk right away."

"What makes you say that babies could talk right away in the olden days?" asked the father.

"Why, we read it in the Bible in Sunday School, said the girl. "We were reading the Book of Job, and it said 'Job cursed the day he was born'!"

Type Faster, Please

As the deadline for his doctoral dissertation approached, a graduate student urged his wife, who was typing for him to hurry up. "The next woman I marry is going to really know how to type," he complained.

"That's all right, dear," she replied. "The next man I marry is going to already have his doctorate."

––––––––

TV Dinner Diet

A lady we know is on a new diet — nothing but TV dinners. She says it helps with her horizontal hold.

––––––––

Traveling Salesman

It was a brutal night. The rain was coming down in sheets. The wind was blowing and visibility was almost nil. The salesman was having trouble driving.

"This is a rough one," he told his pet dog, Fido, who accompanied him on all his trips. "Looks like we're in for it!"

No sooner had he stopped speaking when he spotted a small motel by the roadside. He couldn't have been happier. He drove up and parked in front of the office, picked up his dog, and walked in.

"I'd like a room for the night," he told the proprietor.

"Sorry, mister," said the man. "We're all filled up."

"I could sleep on the sofa," suggested the salesman.

"That's where I sleep."

"But you can't turn me out on a night like this," protested the salesman.

The man at the desk simply shrugged, and the salesman realized it was useless to plead. He turned to go, but the man stopped him before he got to the door.

"Just a minute mister," he said. "Leave the pup here. I wouldn't turn a dog out on a night like this!"

––––––––

Taxi Please

A cab driver noticed a young woman waving frantically at him to pull over. He responded to her request and stopped to let her into his cab. She got into the cab and commented on how she was so pleased that he was kind enough to pick her up.

"Could you please take me to the airport across town so I can catch the twelve o'clock flight to Houston."

"Yes ma'am, I will certainly try," he said, "but you do realize that that gives me only ten minutes?"

"Yes, I know, but please try," she added.

So off they went through the noon traffic. They finally made it to the airport with one minute to spare. The woman got out of the cab, thanked the driver and proceeded to give him a fifteen-cent tip.

"Lady, this fifteen-cent tip is an insult."

"Oh?" she said. "How much should it be?"

"Another fifteen cents, at least," said the driver.

"My dear fellow," she said, "I wouldn't dream of insulting you twice!"

————

Have your helper make up questions about the story once you have understood it.

— Chapter VII —

AUDITORY TRAINING
FOR CHILDREN

W HEN sound is first amplified for the hard-of-hearing child, he is faced with a new or at least a different auditory experience. Sounds that were previously inaudible are now new and strange to the hearing-impaired child. Sounds that were soft, may now be quite loud, but still fuzzy and distorted, or meaningless. Before the child will derive much benefit from amplification, he must be taught to make meaning out of this imperfect sound pattern and supplement what he hears, with what he sees on the lips, in order to develop his language and understanding vocabulary and eventually his speaking vocabulary.

The hearing-impaired child finds that he must rely heavily on his visual and feeling senses in order to learn to communicate with people. If we are to be successful in our auditory training program with children, we must take the auditory information, made available through amplification, and make it an interesting and important ingredient for the development of his total communication skills. Initially, many of the sounds the child hears may seem strange to him and he may be curious, fascinated, confused, or frightened by them. However, after the child has worn the hearing aid for a while and has received auditory training in gross-sound discrimination, the amplified sounds will become more familiar and recognizable to him and he will be able to accept them and place these sounds meaningfully in his auditory world.

The following training lessons, are designed to help the hearing-impaired child adjust properly to his new amplified auditory experiences. These drills should make the new sounds more recognizable and consequently more interesting and useful to his communication effort.

TRAINING THE VERY YOUNG CHILD

Reception and understanding of speech sounds are necessary for the development of speech production. This requires the child to develop fine sound discrimination. Auditory training, however, must develop through a natural progression from gross to fine listening skills. Before the child can learn to speak he must be shown that by listening to noises and, later, sounds, and learning to make them himself, he will be able to develop more and more control over his environment. While we are working on gross-sound discrimination, we should always expose the child to speech that is associated with the toys. Thus, when we are playing gross-sound discrimination games, we should not forget to talk about the objects being used or the tasks being done.

When working with a young hard-of-hearing child, you should begin training by using actual sound-making objects such as bells, horns, whistles, drums, snappers, etc. The child's motivation to learn to recognize things by their sounds will arise from his interest in them as toys in a game or play situation. Four or five noisemakers should be placed on a table in front of the child. First permit the child to become familiar with the training objects, and allow him to examine the noisemakers and play with them. Make a noise with each of the noisemakers several times. Encourage the child to sound each of the noisemakers. If he is reluctant, help him. Then sound one of the noisemakers, and ask by gesture or word, for him to sound the same noisemaker. Then have the child turn his back or close his eyes. Again sound a noisemaker and have the child open his eyes or turn around. Gesture for him and tell him to find the noisemaker which you used. At first, the child will probably require much reinforcement of instruction and much encouragement in doing these tasks.

When the child has become successful at this task, the difficulty can be raised by increasing the number of noisemakers from which the child must choose.

When the child has successfully accomplished the above drills, he is ready for a more advanced gross-sound discrimination drill. You will need two matched sets of four or five similar sounding noisemakers that are slightly different in pitch or quality. These can be made by partially filling small matchboxes or pillboxes with different materials such as "BB" shot, glass beads, small stones, sand, or pennies. Five or six shaker type bells or whistles of similar pitch and quality may also be used. Arrange your set and the child's set of noisemakers on the table so that they are in different order. Sound one of the noisemakers and have the child try to match the sound with a noisemaker from his set. From this level you may progress to a toy xylophone and finally a piano for the sound matching game.

An intermediate drill would be to cut out simple pictures from magazines and paste on cards. It is good to get pictures of objects which have sounds as well as a single name associated with them. Present the card and give the noise associated with the picture and the name. Let the child hold the card, make the noise and take the card from him. Repeat this exercise a number of times; then make the noise; name the card; and extend your hand for the child to give the card to you. Give him several cards which have been used in the previous steps; ask for one by noise; help the child select the card and give it to you. Repeat this task many times. Finally ask for one of the cards by name and extend your hand for the child to give you the correct card. For variation, the above drill can be done using small plastic toy animals and toy representations of real objects which make noise.

A still more advanced drill involves developing better listening habits — beginning speech-sound discrimination and auditory memory for different speech-sound patterns — which allows for better understanding and also better repetition and imitation of speech heard.

The hard-of-hearing young child delayed in language and speech, does not use his auditory perceptive abilities efficiently. Sounds, particularly the complex patterns of speech, do not have adequate meaning to the child and therefore he does not listen very carefully to the spoken voice. He does not discriminate or "separate out" the individual parts and thus fails to retain patterns of speech-sound combinations. This means that the child finds it difficult to learn speech through repetition of ordinary conversation or even from careful speech stimulation. For this next exercise then, select speech sounds that are already within the child's productive ability. This group usually includes the spoken vowels and the bilabial (p,b,m,w) and sometimes the tongue tip (t,d,n) consonants. Remember, this exercise is not trying to teach the child to say new sounds, but only to teach him to attend to the voice carefully and perceive the message accurately and to be able to give the sounds back in exactly the same order in which they were originally given.

Drills should begin with vowels. Any three vowels may be chosen. When the whole series of three vowels has been successfully repeated by the child, one to three other vowels may be substituted for a new series. After success with vowels alone, one of the simple bilabial consonants can be used in front of these same vowels making a more difficult series like; pā, poo, po, or pah, paw, pı̆.

The next order of difficulty would be using different easy consonants used with the same vowels as in pah, mah, tah, or pah, dah. Finally the most difficult listening and repeating task would be combining various easy consonants with various vowels for example tēē, bah, go or pā, mı̄, dah.

When the child is able to repeat accurately these various nonsense syllable combinations in exactly the same order as originally given; he will be able to better separate out spoken sounds. Also he will be able to listen all the way through a word, phrase, or sentence rather than get a fleeting bit at the beginning or end. Thus he can better profit from the speech stimulation which goes on about him every day.

In order to keep his interest and attention and motivate him to want to work with you on these drills, provide a simple reward activity which proves effective for your particular child. This might be drawing a scribbled "picture" on a page or dropping a marble in a box or peg in a board. Competition games to complete the child's or parent's "stick man" or ladder, may also be used.

HELPING THE SCHOOL-AGE CHILD

The hard-of-hearing school-age child will need training to help him recognize and differentiate between the amplified auditory signal and the previously unamplified and perhaps distorted signal. A hard-of-hearing child will find that the speech signal, and speech consonants in particular, will be poorly perceived even with a hearing aid, when it is difficult or impossible to see the speaker's lips. Words, then, will often tend to run together, and instructions by hearing alone will often be garbled and distorted.

Because of this speech discrimination problem, it is imperative that this child be given every opportunity possible to read the speaker's lips to supplement what is gotten from the hearing aid. Parents and teachers can help the hard-of-hearing child by doing the following things:

1. Do not shout if the child is wearing his hearing aid. You are overloading the aid and causing distortion. In addition, the increased loudness may actually be painful.
2. Look directly at the child when you are talking to him.
3. When you talk, do not cover up your mouth with a book, a newspaper, or with your hands.
4. Do not speak with a cigar, a cigarette, or a pipe in your mouth.
5. Hold your head still and steady when speaking.
6. Adjust your position so that the light (whether from a lamp or a window) is on your face, not on the child's face.
7. Speak slowly.
8. Speak distinctly with an active mouth. Do not slur or mumble.
9. If the child fails to get your meaning, rephrase or reword, as well as repeat what you have said.
10. Be patient.
11. Remember that lip reading and listening work together, and one never interferes with the other.
12. Encourage the child to look at the speaker's mouth at all

times so that he sees the lip position of the words as he
hears them.

13. If he is a new hearing aid wearer, help the child to investigate or find the sources of all new sounds. Tell him the
name of the object or animal which is making the sound
as he hears and sees it.

14. After the child has learned to identify sounds, play "eyes-
covered" games in which he must tell you or show you
the sound he heard.

15. Have the child pick up objects as you say the names —
first with watching your lips and listening, and then
with listening alone.

16. Have the child listen to difficult words and word pairs
that sound alike, identifying what he has heard (for example, bat-cat, shoe-two, tie-pie, cap-cup, bed-bread).
Picture cards of these combinations may be made to improve interest and motivation.

17. The listening drill involving combinations of nonsense
syllables described in the previous section, should be used
periodically with the school-age child to make his listening more efficient and improve his discrimination and
auditory memory.

CONCLUSION

This home-training book of speech reading and auditory
training exercises has been devised to help you begin to understand speech better. It is not our intention to provide you with
a complete course in speech reading. Many of you can obtain
further formal training by enrolling in a speech reading course
such as is available at a university or a speech and hearing
center; or, if this is not available to you, you may have further
home-training practice by using a drill book such as "What
People Say" (See Appendix B).

Remember that continual practice is required to maintain
your speech reading and listening abilities. The success of a
rehabilitation program depends upon your acceptance of your
problem, your interest and motivation in overcoming it, and

your willingness to work hard despite occasional discourage-
ments and times of slow progress.

Remember also that learning speech reading is like learning
to play the piano — you never get "finished" with the job. You
just keep getting more and more able to read lips faster and
under adverse conditions such as poor lighting, when the
speaker mumbles with lazy lips, or when he is partially turned
away so you have only a side view of his face.

APPENDICES

INFORMATION SOURCES FOR
THE HARD-OF-HEARING

1. The Alexander Graham Bell
   Association for the Deaf
   3417 Volta Place, N.W.
   Washington, D. C., 20007
   Phone (202) 337-5220

This organization provides information in the form of books, pamphlets, and periodicals on hearing impairment, together with available schools, to students, parents, and the general public. Their Volta Bureau Library is one of the world's largest collections on deafness and is open to all and lends selected publications by mail to members of the Alexander Graham Bell Association. The Bell Association publishes and distributes hundreds of books and pamphlets on hearing and hearing impairment. It publishes the official journal of the Association called "The Volta Review" which reports the latest professional thought on education of the hearing impaired, and provides practical guidance in auditory training and speech reading.

2. American Annals of the Deaf
   Gallaudet College
   Washington, D. C.

Write for the January issue of the magazine which is a complete directory of schools, teachers, religious organizations, camps, publications, teacher-training colleges, clinics, etc., for the deaf and hard-of-hearing in the United States and Canada.

3. Hearing News —

Official publication of the American Hearing Society
817 - 14th Street N.W.
Washington, D. C.

Books and pamphlets on hearing and information regarding a
local chapter are available through the Society.

4. Better Hearing Institute
   1001 Connecticut Ave. N. W.
   Suite 632
   Washington, D. C., 20036

A nonprofit educational organization providing public service,
consumer education, and public information programs for the
hard-of-hearing, their families, and friends.

5. Information Office
   National Institute of Neurological Diseases and Stroke
   National Institute of Health
   U. S. Department of Health, Education and Welfare
   Bethesda, Maryland 20014

Pamphlets available on hearing loss for all ages and education
and training of the preschool deaf child, as well.

6. American Speech and Hearing Association
   9030 Old Georgetown Road
   Washington, D. C., 20014

Order one or both of these publications:

*Guide to Clinical Services in Speech Pathology and Audi-
ology* and *Directory of Members of the Association*

Yearly directories of organizations and individual audiologists
and speech pathologists who can provide assistance and information for the hard-of-hearing in your locality.

7. National Association For Hearing and Speech Action
NAHSA action series of pamphlets on hearing loss and
hearing aids
814 Thayer Ave.
Silver Spring, Maryland 20910

8. John Tracy Clinic
806 W. Adams Blvd.
Los Angeles, California 90007

Appendix B

BIBLIOGRAPHY OF DRILL BOOKS

Speech Reading

1. Broberg, Rose F., *Stories and Games for Easy Lipreading Practice*, 1963.
2. Bunger, Anna M., *Speech Reading, Jena Method*, 1961, Lessons — Adults and Children.
3. Copeland, Medary R., *A Lipreading Practice Manual for Teenagers and Adults*, 1969. Exercises, drills, stories, and discrimination tests.
4. Ewing, Alexander, and Ethel, *Hearing Aids, Lipreading and Clear Speech*, 1967. Practical methods of self-help for the hard of hearing adult.
5. Fisher, Mae T., *Improve Your Lipreading*, 1968. Graded exercises and paragraphs based mainly on visible movements. Excellent practice material for teenagers and adults.
6. Grzebien, Albert E., *Speechreading Through Sports*, 1967. Games, puzzles, exercises for junior high and older football fans.
7. Haspiel, George S., *A Synthetic Approach to Lipreading*, 1964. Graded lessons for children 5-14 yrs.
8. Nitchie, Elizabeth H., *New Lessons in Lipreading*.
9. Ordman, Kathryn A and Ralli, Mary P., *What People Say — The Nitchie School Basic Course in Lipreading*, 1965.
10. Sortini, Adam J., *Speechreading (A Guide for Laymen)*.
11. Whitehurst, M. W., *Integrated Lessons in Lipreading and Auditory Training*, 1964.

Auditory Training

1. Kelly, J. C., *Clinician's Handbook for Auditory Training*, 1973. Drills to improve auditory discrimination and auditory memory for adults and older children.
2. Rubin, Martha, *Our Noisy World*, 1974. An auditory training booklet with 12 illustrated short stories and featuring environmental sounds on cassette tape.
3. Whitehurst, Mary Wood, *Auditory Training for Children*, 1966. Graded lessons from very simple to difficult.
4. Utley, Jean, *What's Its Name?* A workbook and record album for preschool and primary age hearing-impaired children.

The above books may be ordered and purchased from:

> The Alexander Graham Bell
> Association for the Deaf
> 3417 Volta Place N.W.
> Washington, D. C., 20007
> Phone (202) 337-5220

Write for their catalogue of titles and prices.

Appendix C

COMMUNICATION DEVICES FOR THE HEARING IMPAIRED

Telephone Amplifiers

Volume Control Handset
(Amplifies incoming message) Telephone Company Business
  Office

Nu Vox Telephone Amplifier-Cat. #978
Hal-Hen, 36-14 Eleventh St., Long Island City, N.Y. 11106

Aid-A-Phone
Amatronics, 1309 W. Valencia Drive, Fullerton, Calif.

Calitone Telephone Amplifier
M. Calig Company, 5024 Lankershim Blvd., North Holly-
  wood, California

Clarafon Telephone Amplifier
Multione Electronics, Limited, 111 Broadway, New York,
  New York

Tel-Pet (Model LP 505)-Small, portable unit attaches to ear-
  piece of telephone receiver-$12
American Overseas Trading, 4619 South Carrollton Ave.,
  New Orleans, La. 70119

Auxiliary Telephone Receivers

Auxiliary Watchcase Receiver
Telephone Company Business Office

Twinphone
Telephone Dynamics Corporation, 1333 Newbridge Road,
North Bellmore, New York

Switchboard Amplifier

Switchboard Amplifier
Local Telephone Company Business Office

Telephone Ringers

Standard Internal Telephone Bells, (805, 1015, 1610, 2025,
2555, 3220, 4060 cycles per second — different pitched
rings).
Local Telephone Company Business Office

External Telephone Bells (Not enclosed in telephone set,
range from 580 to 1500 cps)
Local Telephone Company Business Office

Extra-strength Gong or Horn
Telephone Company Business Office

Telephone or Doorbell Ringer

Fone-A-Lert battery powered unit emits loud, piercing sound
whenever the telephone or doorbell, to which it is attached
rings.
Hal-Hen Company 36-14 Eleventh St., Long Island City,
New York, 11106

The Bell Telephone System has developed more than a dozen
aids to help make telephoning easier for the hard-of-
hearing, from amplifiers to specially designed sets that
allow people to "see" or "feel" a telephone conversation.
Write for free booklets
"Aids For The Hard of Hearing";
195 Broadway
Room 540, New York, New York 10007

Electronic Switches for installation of individual room signal lights which light along with the telephone ring

> Auxiliary Signal Control — Telephone Company Business Office

> Sign-Trol — Electronics Company, 1949 Coney Island Avenue, Brooklyn, New York

> Automatic Clock Lamps and Vibrators — to awaken you by vibration or bright light

> Time-O-Matic and Digital Moonbeam Flashalarm Clock. Hal-Hen Company, 36-14 Eleventh Street, Long Island City, New York, 11106

> Vibralarm
> Vibralarm Service, 29 Cedar Avenue, Farmingdale, New York
> Vibrating Alarm Clock — Crt. #878 — Hal-Hen Company.

Radio and Television Audio Control Apparatus Write for their descriptive catalogs. (For special Radio and TV miniature speakers and earphones with individual volume controls)

> Adaphone
> Multitone Electronics Limited, 111 Broadway, New York, New York

> Miniature Personalized Speaker
> Wright Zimmerman Incorporated, New Brightin, St. Paul, Minnesota

> Marvel Inductor
> Hal-Hen Company, 36-14 Eleventh Street, Long Island City, New York

> Phonoduct
> Siemens Medical of America, 685 Liberty Avenue, Union, New Jersey

TV Pillow Loudspeakers
Danavox North America, Incorporated, Wayzata, Minnesota

TV Telecom
Noisegard, Incorporated, 2432 Grand Concourse, New York,
New York

Typewritten messages for visual communication over any telephone, with simple battery operated, portable typewriter-like
unit. Ask for the MCM Communications System. Write:

> Micon Industries, Inc.
> 252 Oak Street
> Oakland, California 94607

Baby Awake Alarms — Nu Vox Sentinel Baby Alarm — Cat.
#909
Hal-Hen Company, 36-14 Eleventh Street, Long Island City,
New York, 11106.

INDEX

123